Living with Asthma and Hay Fever

REVISED EDITION

John Donaldson

PENGUIN BOOKS

PENGUIN BOOKS

Published by the Penguin Group
Penguin Books Ltd, 27 Wrights Lane, London W8 5TZ, England
Penguin Books USA Inc., 375 Hudson Street, New York, New York 10014, USA
Penguin Books Australia Ltd, Ringwood, Victoria, Australia
Penguin Books Canada Ltd, 10 Alcorn Avenue, Toronto, Ontario, Canada M4V 3B2
Penguin Books (NZ) Ltd, 182–190 Wairau Road, Auckland 10, New Zealand

Penguin Books Ltd, Registered Offices: Harmondsworth, Middlesex, England

First published 1989
Revised edition 1994
10 9 8 7 6 5 4 3 2 1

The artwork for the figures in this book was drawn by
David Gifford and Capricorn Design

Set in 10.5/13 pt Monotype Bembo
Typeset by Datix International Limited, Bungay, Suffolk
Printed in England by Clays Ltd, St Ives plc

PENGUIN BOOKS

LIVING WITH ASTHMA AND HAY FEVER

After National Service in the Rifle Brigade, John Donaldson read PPE at Christ Church, Oxford, and has made his career in industry including, at one time, the pharmaceutical industry. A lay member of the Management and Education Committees of the National Asthma Campaign (NAC), he writes regularly for *Asthma News*.

COMMENTS ON THE FIRST EDITION (1989)

'The most comprehensive and up-to-date of books on asthma which will be of interest to a wide readership . . . He has succeeded in describing complex theoretical arguments in a simple and readable manner' – Dr Naomi Eiser in *Asthma News*

'I congratulate you on tackling so many simple but important questions. The concept of having such a good book written by a patient is splendid' – Professor Dame Margaret Turner-Warwick, Past President of the Royal College of Physicians and formerly Dean of the Royal Brompton Hospital

'I consider it to be almost in advance of conventional medical management with an excellent chapter on adjusting treatment to suit the illness – this chapter alone justifies purchase of the book' – Dr Martyn Partridge in *Respiratory Disease in Practice*

Contents

PART FOUR *Complementary Medicine*

PART FIVE *Appendices*

List of Figures

Foreword

Nowadays the media are full of the marvels of modern medicine and greet even small discoveries as 'breakthroughs' so that it almost seems strange that anyone is ever ill. It is indeed true that serious illnesses which used to kill many thousands of people every year, such as smallpox, typhoid, cholera, pneumonia and tuberculosis, have been conquered by hygiene, vaccination and antibiotics. But several common ailments remain which, although not yet prevented or cured, can be controlled by powerful remedies discovered by medical science. These succeed, however, only if doctors and patients collaborate closely in their use. Old-fashioned 'doctor's orders' are of little use here. Patients have to learn about their illnesses and understand how their medicines act if they are to be effective.

Asthma and hay fever are typical examples of this situation. Modern treatments are now so powerful that the distressing and occasionally dangerous narrowing of the air tubes in the lungs, which causes difficult breathing, can be overcome by their use in all but a few especially difficult cases. And yet many patients remain disabled by asthma and the number of deaths it causes each year continues to rise.

There seem to be two main reasons for this sorry state of affairs. One is that many doctors, as students, were not taught how to recognize asthma and haven't yet learnt about the new methods of treatment. The other is that some people with asthma seem almost to deny their illness, resent their dependence on health professionals and do not or will not take the trouble to learn about the nature of their asthma and its treatment. Moreover, few doctors are really good at teaching patients or can give time to it.

This is where a book like this one can be so useful. It is written by someone who has had to cope with severe asthma since he was a boy but who has, at meetings of branches of the National Asthma Campaign, not only learnt how to keep his own asthma at bay but also has gone on to acquire a full understanding of the intricate and microscopic reactions in the lungs which cause asthma and how modern medicines can act to stop or reverse them.

If you have asthma, just learning all these details will not by itself ensure that you will manage to control it better. To do that, you have to decide (a) to understand your symptoms, (b) to see whether any of your present ways need changing, and (c) to follow any of the useful suggestions which you will find in these pages and which fit your particular sort of asthma or hay fever. The test of your success will be if you do as John Donaldson has done and have fewer attacks, less wheezing and greater physical activity – studying this book will have been well worth the effort; if you have severe asthma it may even save your life.

Charles Fletcher, C.B.E., M.D., F.R.C.P., F.F.P.H.M.

Preface

Let us imagine that it is a beautiful day in early summer. You decide to take a stroll in the countryside. The birds are singing and you rejoice in the sight and smell of the flowers and the rich smell of newly mown hay; it feels good to be alive. But your joy is short-lived: your eyes begin to itch and stream, sharp needles seem to be at work in your nostrils and you soon feel listless and lethargic. You have hay fever.

On the following day the barometer falls and the weather changes. Storm clouds gather and then there is a squall of rain. You begin to notice that your breathing has become difficult and your chest feels as though a band has been placed round it and is being tightened. You start to cough and splutter; you feel ill-at-ease and a little apprehensive. You have asthma.

Of these two illnesses it is asthma which is the more distressing. It is true that hay fever makes you miserable: you feel as though your head is about to explode and concentration is difficult. But hay fever does not affect your speech or your ability to move around. Very few have died as the result of an attack of hay fever.

Asthma is described as an **inflammation** of the airways, due to the infiltration of white cells. The function of the airways is explained, and the way in which they can become narrowed to a pin-point.

Allergy is a response to **triggers.** These fall into two groups. In the first group are allergens, which are derived from living matter, and virus infections: these tend to make the underlying sensitivity worse and the airways more responsive. The second group of triggers are not allergic, but act as irritants and have a short-term effect.

The **medicines** are arranged in families, with a distinction made between the *relievers* (which reverse an attack) and the *preventers* (which damp down the underlying inflammation). The many kinds of inhaler devices are described.

When choosing the **treatment**, doctors increasingly follow 'The Guidelines'. These are described and illustrated with case histories. There follows a check-list of what to do when things go wrong.

Asthma is a variable illness, and this calls for **self-management** by the patient on a day-to-day basis. Guidance is provided not only by the symptoms but also by readings from a simple peak flow meter, in accordance with treatment plans.

The special problems of managing asthma in **children**, from infancy, are dealt with in the form of answers to the many questions which parents ask. Schooldays and holidays present additional challenges.

While asthma in children is typically episodic and fully reversible, in **adults** it tends to be more persistent and less easy to reverse. This can interfere with work, especially if there are harmful chemicals which trigger the illness. Exercise can be a problem.

Food allergy is not a common cause of asthma but it concerns mothers in particular. The foods which can act as triggers are examined.

Hay fever (or, rather, rhinitis in various forms) affects the nose and eyes, and sometimes hearing as well, and has the same triggers as asthma and similar cell responses. New treatments are available and these are fully described, especially those aiming at prevention.

The way we confront any illness is powerfully influenced by the **response of others**, be they carers, friends, colleagues or health professionals. Asthma, in particular, is generally misunderstood by lay people and this has unfortunate consequences. Welfare services are reluctant providers of support when an illness is variable.

This helps to explain the recent growth of **voluntary organizations**, such as the National Asthma Campaign, and the increasing attention that is being paid to the training of community nurses in the appropriate skills.

It also explains a growing interest, albeit by a small minority of patients, in **alternative medicine**. This is not generally supported by scientific evidence, but it does at least pay detailed attention to the patient as an individual.

Finally, the book is designed both as a continuous narrative and also as a **work of reference**. This has led to some unavoidable repetition, because each section is designed to stand alone. An up-to-date reading-list is provided together with useful addresses and an index; and 'The Questions People Ask' will prove useful in an emergency. It is a good idea to read Chapter One first!

The text is appropriate throughout the English-speaking world since it incorporates guidelines for the management of asthma which are now accepted internationally. Both generic and brand names are given for the medicines, and local brands are listed where known. Technical terms are avoided wherever possible and are explained where they first occur.

My viewpoint is that of someone who has received most of the treatments for both asthma and hay fever of varying degrees of severity. My aim in writing the book has been at every stage to introduce the problems encountered by families with an asthmatic member and to draw on high authorities for the answers. 'Happy is he who can understand the causes of things.'

John Donaldson
Fulham, May 1994

Acknowledgements

In the first edition of *Living with Asthma and Hay Fever* I acknowledged the help received from the many talks on asthma and hay fever given to branches of the National Asthma Campaign by specialists in the London area. I also drew on the course devised by the Asthma Training Centre and publications by the National Asthma Campaign. Certain chapters were checked by doctors with special knowledge and the manuscript as a whole was read by Dr John Rees, Senior Lecturer at Guy's Hospital. Professor Charles Fletcher kindly provided a Foreword, which is retained.

This second edition is a complete revision, taking into account many developments since 1989. Once again the pharmaceutical companies have helped with up-to-date information (Allen and Hanburys, Astra Pharmaceuticals, Fisons Pharmaceuticals, 3M Health Care and Napp Laboratories). Special thanks are due to Professor Richard Beasley of the Wellington School of Medicine, New Zealand, for comments on the chapter on self-management; to Dr Jonathan Dare of King's College Hospital, London, for reading the chapter on the human response; to Dr Michael Silverman of the Hammersmith Hospital, London, for looking over the chapter on asthma in children; and to Dr Derek Williams of St Mary's Hospital, Paddington, for reviewing the chapter on hay fever. The text as a whole has greatly benefited from comments by Dr Bill Frankland, Honorary Consultant Allergist to Guy's Hospital.

I am grateful to my editor, Eleo Gordon, and copy-editor, Roger Wells, for converting an untidy manuscript into the present book.

PART ONE

Living with Asthma

CHAPTER ONE

Living with Asthma

Introduction

Most people take each breath for granted – which is not surprising, since it arrives about 1,800 times every hour! But this is not always possible for those of us who have asthma.

Even mild asthma can be disturbing. It may take the form of coughing, or breathlessness, or (less commonly) wheezing, or even all three combined. If the attacks persist, the family is likely to be as concerned as the patient but at a loss to know how to help, and I have written this book with carers very much in mind.

With their great vitality, children are resilient and tend to forget, in between attacks, that they are at risk. But older people, with their more persistent asthma, may find that it changes their whole way of life. It was sad to receive a letter from an elderly lady who wrote: 'I don't go out that much because the attacks can come on so quickly and people don't know how to help me.'

Quite a common illness

It is surprising to people with asthma, who can feel rather isolated, to learn that it affects at least one child in ten. Asthma can start at any age, from early infancy to the eighties. It often appears in early childhood, disappears at puberty or the late teens and then remains hidden until, in about 5 per cent of all adults, it reappears in later life. Up to the time of adolescence it is twice as common in boys as in girls; after that, girls are equally likely to have it.

The improvements in treatments

In the past there were many strange treatments for asthma, not to mention the disturbing side-effects from remedies such as adrenaline, ephedrine and isoprenaline. Nowadays the medicines are so effective that most people with asthma, if properly treated, can live full and active lives for most of the time. Even when taken on a daily basis, the new medicines are safe in that any side-effects will be short-lived.

Fifty years ago asthma meant days in bed, propped up against pillows. Nowadays children with asthma can take part in games and sports and are as likely as other children to compete successfully in competitions. Some older people with asthma have to adjust their lives to the illness but, unless the asthma is very severe, they can remain mobile and active even though the asthma is present all the time.

As recently as the 1970s all that the medicines aimed to do was to reverse an attack already under way. Now we have in addition treatments which can prevent an attack from taking place. One of the aims of the new treatments is to damp down 'twitchiness' in the airways, so that they are less likely to respond to one of the many triggers that can provoke an attack to take place. The medicines will be fully described in Chapter Four.

Asthma is often poorly controlled

In spite of the improved medicines, asthma is still poorly controlled in many families. This is borne out by recent surveys and the too numerous admissions to hospitals. Asthma is responsible for more schooldays lost than any other illness and is the cause of millions of man-hours being lost through absence from work. Asthma is the only treatable illness in Western civilization that is on the increase; for example, in 12-year-old children studied in Cardiff the proportion with asthma (and hay fever) doubled from 1973 to 1988.

What are the reasons for this lamentable state of affairs? It may well be that changes in the environment (which will be examined in Chapter Three) have made asthma more prevalent, so the medicines have to work harder.

Most people approach the treatments with caution. Some remember the side-effects resulting from high doses of tablet steroids when they were introduced in the 1950s; nowadays routine treatment is with *inhaled* steroids and safety is the key-note. Patients may well be confused when *anabolic* steroids are mentioned in the press; these are never used in the treatment of asthma or hay fever.

The word 'drug' itself, though it applies to any ingredient used in the pharmacy, has always had sinister overtones and brings to mind such problems as addiction and drug abuse. It happens that not one of the medicines used in asthma is addictive. But we all have a natural reluctance to take any kind of medicine on a daily basis.

Myths have gathered round the illness, and these can stand in the way of successful treatment. It is a widely held belief that asthma is 'psychosomatic': a kind of nervous disorder; this view is not shared by chest physicians. Children sometimes worry whether it is 'catching'; it is not infectious. Not a few parents worry that it may be a life sentence which will condemn their child to a permanent state of physical inferiority. That this is far from being the case is proved by the fact that many world-class athletes, in a variety of sports and games, have asthma or suffered in childhood from it.

The role of the doctor

Patients who are critical of their doctor complain that he or she does not listen to their problems, does not explain the treatments, skates over the side-effects and is not at all concerned about measures to reduce the possible triggers in the home. Patients often feel that the messages are 'robotic' and standardized. They become confused when a change of doctor brings a change of treatment, sometimes accompanied by disparaging remarks about what was given previously. They do not understand why only a few tablets are prescribed so that they have to return to the surgery even when unwell, to plead for a replenishment.

In their turn, doctors complain that patients absorb very little information; that they rely too much on the relieving medicines but at the same time do not take the preventing medicines as prescribed. Patients get used to the symptoms of asthma and as a result expect less from the treatments than they should deliver. Patients go along too readily with the idea that all illness is due to external causes, beyond their control, and that asthma is the kind of illness you should learn to live with, so they make the least fuss possible. After a time they forget what a normal airway feels like and adapt their lives to suit the illness to an excessive degree.

Some patients angrily or fearfully reject the notion that they have asthma and refuse to take a remedy. As a result, some doctors, when confronted with a wheezy chest, avoid the word 'asthma' and use instead a label such as 'wheezy bronchitis'. This may be less alarming for the patient but it could lead to under-prescribing or using the wrong drugs.

A variable illness

Another reason why asthma may be poorly controlled is that the attacks can arrive suddenly and without much warning: they are hard to predict because the triggers which provoke them are constantly changing. The result is that the medicines are not taken in time, or at an appropriate level of dosage, or they are switched off as soon as the symptoms fade with the result that the asthma soon reasserts itself.

As Professor Fletcher observed in his Foreword, authoritarian 'doctor's orders' are of little use in the shifting world of the asthmatic, and the patient has to learn, slowly and painfully, how to become an asthma specialist, able to adapt the treatments to each twist and turn of the illness.

This kind of self-knowledge, and skill in self-management, can only be acquired gradually, on a step-by-step basis. Only fragments can be picked up in a traditional six-minute medical consultation. This is why I have designed this book to be used as a kind of primer, with concepts introduced in stages, as well as being accessible as a reference book.

What is asthma?

The word 'asthma' has come down to us from the Greeks and simply means 'to breathe hard'. Breathlessness, wheezing and coughing may all suggest the presence of asthma, but this is not exclusively so, since they can be produced by other illnesses.

The *coughing* occurs because the airways become inflamed and sensitive; there is *shortness of breath* because the lungs have to work harder to obtain enough oxygen; *wheezing* is less common but is due to the passage of air through narrowed breathing tubes. The last symptom can be demonstrated to children by allowing air to escape through the twisted neck of a balloon.

The most distinctive characteristic of asthma has already been mentioned: the symptoms constantly vary, as between daytime and night-time, from one season to another, and according to the many triggers which can provoke the attacks. These may be separated by long intervals of time, which can be counted in months or even years, or they may occur very frequently, typically on a seasonal basis. In 'chronic' (that is, *persistent*) asthma, the symptoms would be continuous if they were not prevented by treatment.

Sometimes the attacks arrive without warning; at other times there are signs – such as listlessness and irritability, a disinclination to eat, and a kind of unease – that the air passages are at risk. Sometimes there is a tingling sensation in the nose and on the skin. Asthma has been compared to a river slowly descending towards the sea until it meets a cliff or escarpment, and then it tumbles headlong downwards.

It will be explained that asthma causes a narrowing of the airways by inflammation (thickening) of the airway tissues; a tightening of the airway muscles and an increase in the output of sticky mucus within the airways. It is when all three combine that a severe attack takes place.

An attack may last for only an hour or so and then clear of its own accord. This is when the muscles alone are involved, for example after a short period of physical exertion. More often it persists, as happens when asthma is triggered by a cold in the head or by an 'allergen' such as pollen, and it can go on for a day or two, or for weeks if not treated with medicines.

What does it feel like?

It is impossible to convey to someone who has never had asthma what an attack feels like. In mild asthma the chest feels tight and it is like breathing through a bent straw. In severe asthma it is more like choking in a room full of smoke. It is not generally recorded in the textbooks that it is a common experience that severe asthma is accompanied by profuse sweating, by a loosening of the bowels and by a feeling of malaise or menace. Energy seems to seep away during an attack because, as we shall see, the body gets short of oxygen and vital organs such as the brain and the heart become tired, so you feel listless. If you have a cold at the same time, this will add to the lassitude.

In young children the main symptom may be a persistent cough which carries on, night after night, until both the parents and child are exhausted. This is not, in spite of the nagging persistence of the cough, a dangerous form of the illness.

It often happens, in children and adults alike, that asthma is worse at night, for reasons which are examined on page 76. Loss of sleep leads to tiredness and irritability during the following day. We are reluctant to summon help at night-time, and when we consult the doctor the next day no vestiges of the illness may remain nor indeed signs of any illness. It is not surprising that we tend to play down symptoms which cannot be reproduced on demand or that some inexperienced doctors dismiss the illness as trivial.

Not one cause, but many

It is often not easy – or even possible – to decide at any given moment which triggers are chiefly responsible for the attacks. We often think we can pinpoint the causes, but we may be mistaken. In recent years it has become fashionable to attribute asthma, hay fever and food illness mainly to 'allergens', invisible particles derived from living matter which upset only those who are 'allergic'.

Bookshops are full of paperbacks which tell us how to avoid these unseen triggers, and they are especially keen to persuade us to change our diet. As we shall see in Chapter Eleven, diet plays only a small part in most people's asthma. In the past we were asked to undergo simple skin scratch tests to discover our particular allergic triggers. These may include house dust, animals, pollens and mould spores.

However there are, in addition, many other triggers which are not strictly allergens, for example breathing in cold or dry air, catching a cold, or being exposed to chemical fumes. It is possible to have asthma without showing any allergic reactions when tested.

The 'friendly' air we breathe turns out to be hostile. At any moment there are likely to be not just a few triggers but many, not only the pollens and house dust but also chemical irritants such as cigarette smoke, fumes from factories and smoke from power stations.

My home in Fulham is close to the old power station which provides electricity for the London Underground. I live in hope that the wind will stay mainly in the south-west and not back eastwards so that it covers the house with chemicals from the station.

Even people's emotional responses can fire an attack: the sharp intake of air during laughter can upset those very sensitive airways. Exercise puts us at risk. Cold air is especially likely to upset older people with asthma, in my own case when moving from a warm room to one which is cooler. The triggers do not work in isolation but can reinforce one another. Sometimes it is the allergen which primes the whole delicate mechanism and an irritant which provokes the reaction. 'Cross-reactivity' takes place: becoming sensitive to one trigger leads to sensitivity to another.

A few people with asthma are very specific in their reaction. They wheeze only when they meet a cat, or eat shellfish, or sleep on a feather pillow. Such people can take avoiding action. For most of us, the air we breathe contains many unseen enemies to which our exquisitely sensitive airways can respond.

Asthma can be dangerous

Deaths from asthma are rare. At the time of writing there are in the United Kingdom about 2,000 deaths a year in a population of about three million people with asthma. Two-thirds of the deaths are in people aged over 65, and this may at least partly account for a period in which the death rate has been rising, since older people are living longer.

The death rate is now stable in this country, in spite of a steady increase in the numbers of people confirmed as having asthma. It seems that the 'environment' in its widest sense is becoming more hostile for people with asthma and this is leading to a higher incidence. On the other hand, the medicines are constantly being improved and we are becoming more skilled in using them.

In this population about 35 children die from asthma each year. It is generally accepted that most asthma deaths could be avoided, given the appropriate emergency treatment. Few deaths take place in hospital; most of them occur at home or when being rushed to the emergency ward. As a mother whose teenage daughter died on the way to hospital explained:

> If only I had known that asthma could be fatal, my daughter might still be alive. No one had told me that a seemingly mild attack could escalate so quickly.

As the quotation suggests, a severe attack can happen suddenly and with little warning. A fatal attack generally occurs between two and five hours after the onset; it follows that any severe attack of asthma should be taken very seriously.

Deaths are not caused by heart failure arising from a strain on the heart, as is commonly supposed, but are due to the sharp reduction in the supply of oxygen to all parts of the body, especially to the brain. This lack of oxygen is shown in a developing blueness of the tongue, lips and nails, and the next stage is a gradual loss of consciousness.

Pains in the chest

It is natural to suppose that, when pain is felt in the chest during an attack of asthma, it is due to a heart attack. This is rare, except in people who have heart disease. The more likely reason is that during an asthma attack the lungs expand because air gets trapped inside them. This stretches the membranes which surround the lungs, the walls of the chest, the rib muscles and diaphragm, and any one of these consequences may result in pain, sometimes described by children as 'tummy pain'.

People with asthma also enquire whether high altitudes are safe, for example when climbing or skiing. In general they feel better in the clean mountain air, but it is thinner and extra puffs from a relieving inhaler may be needed.

Asthma in times past

It is tempting to suppose that asthma is solely a by-product of modern civilization: of polluted air, of chemicals in our food, of crowded travel and workplaces where germs are exchanged; or that it is made worse by urban stress and strain.

This is not so. As Dr Alex Sakula reminded us in a fascinating paper tracing the history of asthma, the ancient Egyptians referred to it in their writings on papyrus and treated the illness not only with the excrement of crocodiles – which we might reject – but also with an inhalation from herbs, such as henbane thrown on to hot bricks. The Chinese wrote about asthma as long ago as 1,000 B.C., at which time they were using a cough linctus made from a plant from which, in modern times, ephedrine has been extracted.

In India, herbs were used 1,500 years ago (as they still are today in Ayurvedic medicine); one of these was introduced into England in the present century by doctors who had served in the Indian Army. One of these Indian herbs contained stramonium, and this turned up in 'Potter's Asthma Cure'. I was treated by it in childhood, watching with fascination as the white powder was set on fire. I can still recall its sharp aroma, rather like snuff. Then, at the age of ten, I had to smoke herbal cigarettes rolled in black paper with a gold band. They were foul and put me off smoking for life!

The Ancient Greeks knew asthma well and thought it was brought about by the 'humours' being out of balance. Their treatment was an emetic together with dieting, or relaxation induced by sedatives, massage, hydrotherapy and auto-suggestion. They were aware that asthma is made worse by exercise and cold air, that it is highly variable and often increases during a period of sleep.

Some remote people are free from asthma

It seems that asthma is quite rare in the rural communities of the Gambia, in West Africa, but is common in neighbouring towns. When a southern Pacific island community had to be evacuated to a mainland city, the incidence of asthma in children doubled. Asthma has increased in Papua New Guinea since Westerners started to move in and provide the natives with mite-infested mattresses.

Various theories have been advanced to explain this spread of asthma. One is that breast feeding is more common in remote rural areas than in urban communities. (This theory does not explain why, in England, children of West Indian and Caucasian families are equally likely to be atopic,* as measured by skin prick tests, yet breast feeding is much more common among the West Indians.) Another theory is that when people move into the towns they eat more complex foods which contain additives of various kinds, and that the additives are to blame. This theory comes up against the fact that in modern Japan there is a low incidence of asthma. Studies at the Hammersmith Hospital in London have shown that children from Indian immigrant families are especially likely to develop allergies to certain Western-type drinks and foods: could this be due to the change in diet rather than to its nature? Dr Duncan Geddes has quoted Gandhi's comment on Western civilization: 'It would be a good idea!'

* 'Atopic', literally 'out of place' (referring to the reaction rather than the trigger), is the clinical term for the allergic condition which can be responsible for asthma and hay fever. Tests for atopy are described on page 55.

Asthma may have links with social class

There is some evidence that children with many brothers and sisters catch colds at an early age from their siblings. This helps them to perfect their immune system, so they become less likely to develop allergic diseases. Large families are most common among the poorer classes.

Children born in families which contain smokers are more likely to suffer from asthma, and old, poor, damp housing may contribute as well, especially if there is a lot of air pollution from factories and vehicles.

It is presumably easier to *tolerate* asthma if you have an office job rather than one which involves exposure to cold or polluted air; however I recall working in an office with a poor air-conditioning system and being more or less permanently 'out of sorts'. 'Occupational asthma' is covered on page 203.

CHAPTER TWO

Why Some People Have Asthma

A difficult question

As a child, I often used to ask myself this question. What had I done to deserve this penalty which at times so diminished the joy of living? The answer may be either simple or exceedingly complicated, depending on how deeply we try to penetrate the mysteries of lung behaviour. It is quite possible to control the illness without bothering at all about the physiology; indeed the question has no final answer and continues to puzzle scientists who spend their lives trying to supply one.

To understand why some people get asthma, it is necessary to start from a definition of what it is. The following definition, by Professor Tim Clark, will set the scene for what follows:

> Asthma is breathlessness caused by a spasm in the muscle of the airways which connect the mouth and throat to the lungs. When this muscle goes into spasm it narrows the airways, obstructs the flow of air, and prevents your lungs from efficiently passing oxygen to the bloodstream and removing carbon dioxide from it.

If asked to describe the lungs, many will answer, rather vaguely, that they are 'a kind of bellows'. We will have to do a little better than this; but first of all we should really start by considering the nose. Whatever its shape or beauty, and however great or small, it acts as a most efficient air filter, managing to take out about 95 per cent of the dust and germs from the air passing through it. It achieves this because the air enters the nasal passages through a narrow aperture and thus becomes turbulent. The air is then thrown against **mucus**, the sticky coating which lines all the nasal passages, including the sinuses. Minute hair-like protuberances called **cilia** sweep away the old mucus, which is continually replenished. The cilia are in constant motion, like a field of corn ruffled by a breeze. If we breathe through our mouths, this cleaning and conditioning do not take place. The mucus also makes the air moist (98 per cent relative humidity) and warm (32°C) and so prepares it for the next stage of its journey.

The air then passes through holes in the back of the nose and enters the throat (the pharynx). This area also takes in food; it then divides into two separate tubes. One tube is the food pipe (oesophagus); this can be closed by a trap-door, which prevents us from inhaling food. The second tube is the windpipe (trachea); you can feel it if you place your thumb and forefinger just below your 'Adam's apple'. The trachea receives air from the throat and continues the cleaning process. It too is covered with sticky mucus, which is propelled upwards and outwards by the cilia, so we can either cough up the dirt and germs that get past the defences in our nose or swallow them and thus render them harmless.

The trachea is the gateway into the lungs. It divides into two passages; one leads to the left lung, the other to the right lung. These air passages are known as the **main bronchi** (we will examine this last word again, in greater detail, when we look at the 'bronchodilators'). The bronchi then divide like the branches of a tree; they divide again and again, getting smaller and smaller, until they reach an internal diameter of about ten microns.*

This may be hard to visualize, but coincidentally it means that the smallest bronchi have the same width as the thickness of a piece of cotton sewing thread. At this stage the bronchi are

* A micron is one-thousandth of a millimetre.

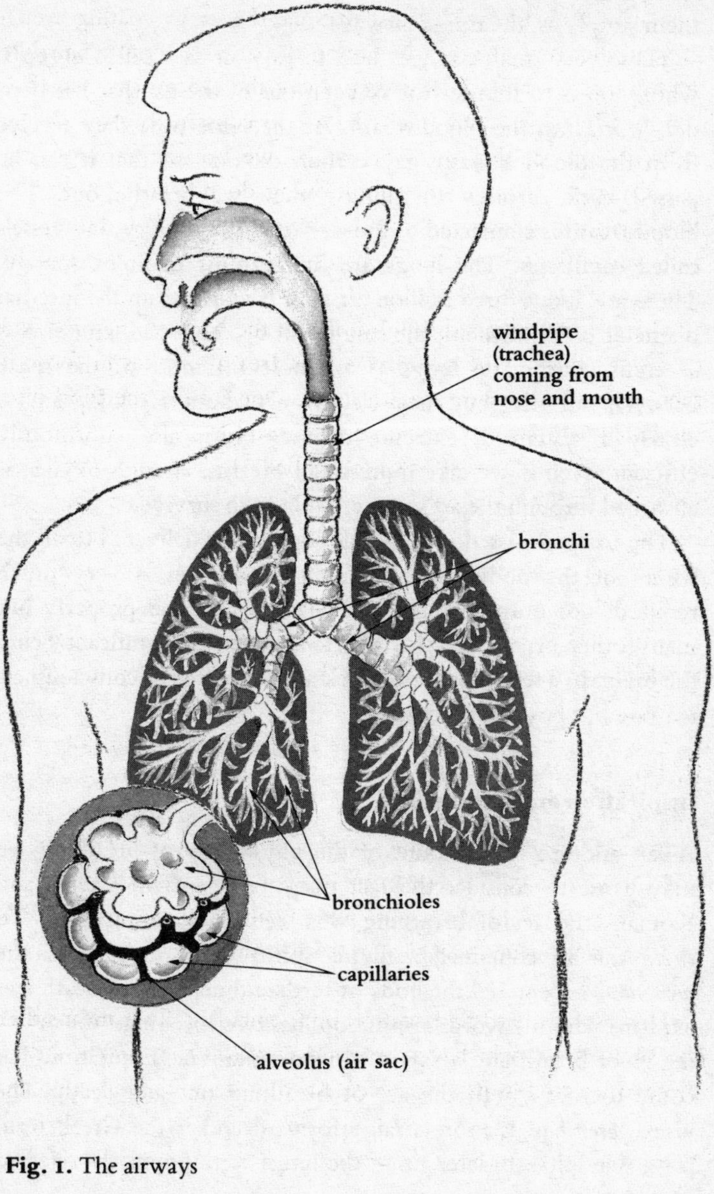

Fig. 1. The airways

known as the **bronchioles** – but it may be easier to refer to them simply as 'the tiniest airways'.

These very small passages lead to tiny air sacs called **alveoli**, whose job is to transfer the oxygen out of the air that has been drawn in, into the bloodstream. At the same time they receive from the blood a waste gas, carbon dioxide, so that it can be passed back through the lungs when we breathe out. The bloodstream is connected to the air sacs through very tiny vessels called capillaries. The lungs are like a most complex sponge. There are about three million air sacs; if you add up the internal diameter of all of them, the result will be about the same size as a tennis court. The lungs as a whole fill most of the space between our ribs, but they weigh only about 1.5 kilograms – clearly a system of extreme delicacy. It is also enormously efficient: even if we take quite small breaths, enough oxygen is absorbed through the air sacs to enable us to survive.

The oxygen passed into the bloodstream is delivered to all the tissues of the body. If the supply of oxygen is very much reduced, not only does the heart fail to function properly but many other organs are also affected, the most significant being the brain. In a severe asthma attack a gradual loss of consciousness is a rare but possible outcome.

Inspiration and expiration

As an aside to this account of the physiology of breathing we may pause to consider the fact that to the ancient Greeks and Romans the act of breathing was seen to be miraculous. To them the air contained a divine spirit which they called the *pneuma*. This entered the body at birth and departed at death and explains why the word 'inspiration' has two meanings: the drawing in of breath and a sort of divine visitation. 'Expiration' has come to mean both the act of breathing out and death. The word '*bronchus*' is more straightforward and is the Greek term for a windpipe. In later times the lungs were popularly referred

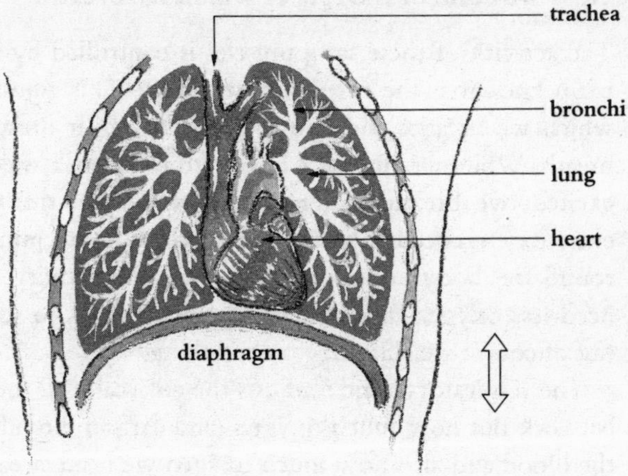

Fig. 2. The diaphragm

to as 'the lights'; this is because, when filled with air after birth, they can float in water!

People with asthma are sensitive to changes in barometric pressure. It is not generally realized that the atmosphere exerts a tremendous pressure on our bodies. Without this pressure, air would not enter the lungs, the blood would burst from its vessels and the body's internal gases would expand alarmingly.

During **inspiration** the cavity in which the lungs have their place increases through the efforts of two kinds of muscles: the ribs are raised like bucket handles and the diaphragm (which lies between the ribs and directly under the lungs) moves downwards like a piston. The empty space so created in the **pleural cavity** is filled with air rushing into the lungs and expanding them. During **expiration** the muscles simply relax and expiration is achieved. The lungs return to their original size.

How we control the rate at which we breathe

The activity of these lung muscles is controlled by a part of the brain known as the **respiratory centre**. This adjusts the rate at which we breathe and also the amount of air drawn in at each breath. When we run for a bus or go for a brisk walk or become excited, we breathe faster and more deeply; this provides the extra oxygen needed by the heart, which has to pump the blood round the body at a rate which suits the activity. In sleep we need less oxygen, and the air machine relaxes to some extent – but of course we still carry on breathing.

The respiratory centre adjusts the air intake all the time. It has to work out how much oxygen (and carbon dioxide) there is in the blood and also how much oxygen we need at each moment. This goes on about 40,000 times every twenty-four hours without any conscious control on our part; it is 'involuntary'. For most of the time we take breathing for granted; we become aware of it only when it becomes laboured: when we climb a mountain, or catch a whiff of smoke from a fire, or suffer an attack of asthma. In these situations we can usually intervene and control the lung muscles: we can decide to breathe more slowly or more deeply. But in a very severe asthma attack we lose this control. Breathing becomes rapid, shallow and automatic, however hard we may try to breathe more deeply. We may even have so little breath that we cannot speak.

What happens during an attack

Anyone exposed to strong fumes, to a thick cloud of dust or to the smoke from a bonfire is likely to cough and choke and bring up mucus. The mucus, or phlegm, is there to protect the delicate linings of the air passages and is part of the mechanism we all have for removing offending particles.

People who are asthmatic respond not only to these overwhelming triggers but also to very small inhalations of dust, smoke or pollen which would not affect their non-asthmatic friends in any way. It is not simply a question of bringing up more mucus. Some asthmatics produce very little and are therefore said to be 'dry'. More significantly, the muscles which surround the air passages in the lungs react by tightening, so the air passages are constricted. The effect is rather like trying to drink through a straw which has collapsed. In addition, the tissues surrounding the airways may become swollen, in much the same way as our skin may become inflamed after an insect bite.

The end result on our breathing tubes of all these actions – the extra mucus, the tightening of the muscles and the swelling of the tissues – is that the passage of air through them becomes difficult. This results in wheeziness and, since the action is likely to take place in many parts of the lungs at the same time, a difficulty in breathing.

A closer look at the air passages

Wheeziness is like the pursing of the lips when we whistle, or allowing air to escape through the neck of an inflated balloon. These analogies are quite helpful, but they may lead us to think of the breathing tubes as if they were like the inner tube of a bicycle tyre or a collapsible toothpaste tube, imagining something resembling a single layer of tough rubber or plastic. What the scientist sees, when he studies a section from one of the air passages through a powerful microscope, is much more complicated:

- on the outside, a band of muscle
- then a layer of connective tissue
- then 'mucosa' (glands which secrete sticky mucus)
- then an inner lining (epithelium)
- attached to this the cilia

The diagram on page 22 will enable us to look at the components of asthma in a little more detail.

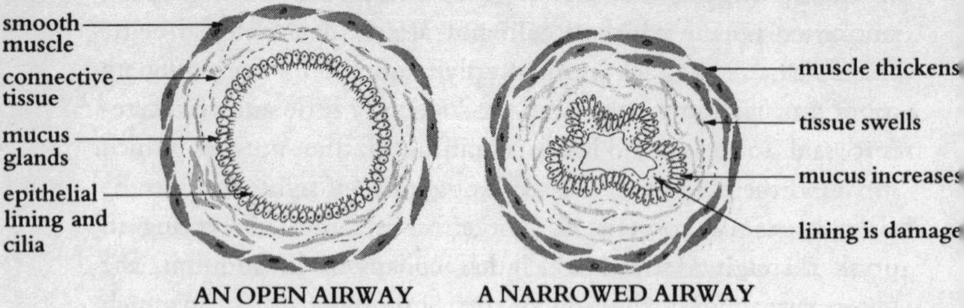

Fig. 3. Cross-section of an airway

Muscle spasm

In most attacks of asthma, the band of muscle which surrounds the air passages thickens, narrowing the aperture. This action is 'involuntary': we cannot control it consciously in the way that we can control the muscles in our hands. To use a medical term, there is **bronchospasm** or **broncho-constriction**. This can take place very rapidly, in both the large and the small air passages, but it rarely occurs in all the passages at the same time, so we are able to continue drawing adequate amounts of air.

The sound of wheezing is caused by spasm or a thickening in *large* air passages, such as the windpipe. (Movement of air through the smallest airways is much slower and, even when they are narrowed, this does not cause wheeziness.)

It is not understood why the muscles go into spasm, since this does not appear to serve any useful function. A similar tightening occurs when we cough, in order to increase the rate of air flow needed to expel the mucus. But this is needed only in the larger breathing tubes, whereas spasm can affect the tiny ones as well.

Inflammation

This is the way our bodies respond to an attack by an invader. For example, if we cut a finger and there is infection, white blood cells invade the tissues in vast numbers, having been transported by the network of blood vessels. The vascular cells (blood cells), which are normally half empty, fill with blood, and as a result the tissues swell. A similar phenomenon further narrows the airways, and it can take place rapidly.

A glance at Figure 3 will show at once that, if the tissues become inflamed, a quite small increase in the thickness of the airway muscles will produce a much bigger reduction in the size of the airway. It has been discovered quite recently that even in mild asthma there is some inflammation even when there are no symptoms, and this is why anti-inflammatory medicines are now prescribed so frequently.

Sticky mucus

We have already mentioned the mucosal glands in the air passages and their ability to secrete sticky phlegm or mucus. In attacks of asthma this can be poured forth in much larger amounts than is normal. The mucus is not necessarily infected (although this can be a possibility), but the debris of dead cells that have perished during their invasion is mixed with it so that, when the airway muscles go into spasm, they can squeeze this mucus into a thin sticky rope. This is hard to dislodge, especially as none of the drugs used in asthma has much effect in thinning it.

Leaky airway linings

Even in mild asthma the thin inner lining of the airways, the **epithelium** (see Figure 3), can become leaky and allow irritants to pass through it and reach the nerve endings which lie just beneath the surface. These nerves can send signals to the airway muscles, which then contract (go into spasm). In a severe attack of asthma the epithelial lining breaks down, adding to the debris and knocking out the cilia which are attached to the epithelium and which are attempting to clear it.

How do we survive a severe attack?

The way a severe attack develops if unchecked with medicines is set out in the form of a table on page 199 in Chapter Ten. Few attacks take the full course shown in this diagram and almost all can be controlled at various stages by using the medicines appropriately.

It may be asked how the body manages to take in enough oxygen when an attack is under way. One explanation is that the airways are affected patchily. It should also be borne in mind that when we breath normally we use only half the capacity of the lungs. By taking a deep breath inwards, we can double this capacity.

Those of us who have asthma learn to compensate for our illness by inflating our rib cages and lowering our diaphragms; when we cannot breathe more deeply, we breathe faster, in proportion to the severity of the attack. Furthermore, we learn to reduce the volume of inspired air which is needed, by resting. When we walk, we take in twice the volume of air compared with what is needed when we are sitting down.

Allergy as a cause of asthma

So far we have looked at what happens in asthma but not at the triggers which can initiate an attack. Chief among these, at least in childhood asthma, are the **allergens**. This word is sometimes used to embrace all the triggers which can be inhaled, but here we restrict its use to those which are of plant or animal origin and which show up on skin prick tests (see page 55).

Allergy has been defined as a state 'in which you are abnormally sensitive to a particular substance'. This abnormal sensitivity can make you feel itchy, it can make your eyes water, or you can feel sick – or it may make you wheezy. The symptoms may occur in the skin (causing eczema or urticaria), in the bowels (leading to diarrhoea), in the nose (causing hay fever) or in the airways of the lungs (producing asthma).

As we shall see in the next chapter, the allergens, in the narrow sense, are referred to as 'specific' triggers. They are mostly proteins and they may arise from dead as well as from live animals or plants; from textiles as well as from cats. Common allergens include:

- the faeces of the house dust mite (which likes to live in pillows, duvets, mattresses and soft furnishings)
- pollen from trees, flowers and grasses (especially in spring and summer), and mould spores
- dandruff and saliva from domestic animals
- some foods (especially milk, eggs, and yeast, in young children)

In infants the most common cause of asthma is not allergy but a virus infection. In children up to the teenage years, house dust mites and pets play an important role, then pollens and moulds take over as the main triggers. In adults, especially those over 45 years old, the most common triggers are not allergens but infections and irritants of chemical origin; also cold air. This is a simplification: both allergens and non-specific irritants are likely to be present in some degree when there is asthma.

Pollen grains and mast cells

To understand more fully the allergic response in asthma, let us take the example of a pollen grain. In early summer there can be a cloud of pollen. Most of it is filtered out by the nose, but a small proportion manages to enter the larger breathing tubes in the lungs. The lining of these tubes is thin, and if it is leaky particles released by the pollen grain will be able to penetrate the airway tissues. **Antibodies** are then summoned to the scene, and in atopic people these arrive in large numbers.

What happens next will be more easily understood if we refer

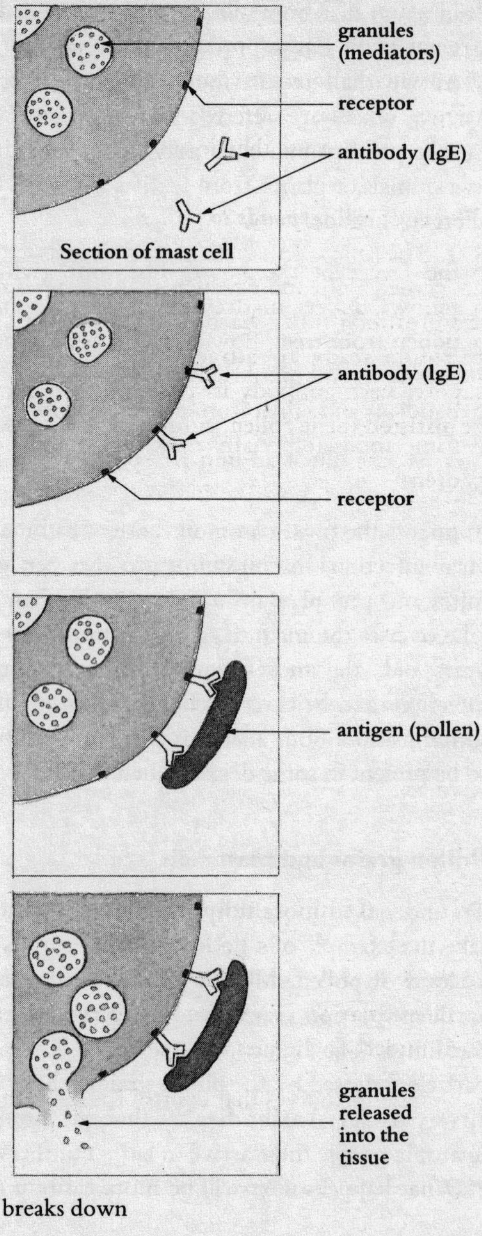

Fig. 4. The mast cell breaks down

to Figure 4. The antibodies lock into **mast cells** which are present in the tissues of the airways. These are now primed so that, when the next invasion of pollen takes place, the antibodies trigger the mast cells, which then release chemicals known as 'mediators' because they initiate a number of responses.

The mast cell responds to pollen

1 The mast cells are widely distributed, but here we are concerned with those which make their home in the linings of the breathing tubes. Each tiny mast cell has up to half a million receptors ready to attract IgE* **antibodies** from the blood supply. Each antibody is specific to a particular kind of trigger, or **antigen** (be it pollen, animals or the house dust mite).

2 As a result of an initial response to an intake of an antigen (such as pollen) into the lungs, the IgE 'pitchforks' lock into an appropriate receptor on the mast cell. The mechanism is now 'primed', but as yet no symptoms are experienced.

3 A few hours, days or weeks later, there is another exposure to this same antigen (i.e. more pollen) and this now forms a bridge across two IgE pitchforks and the result is that the mast cell leaks or quickly releases its packets of poison, a store of granules (chemical **mediators** such as histamine, leukotriene, and prostaglandins).

The role of histamine

The way this procedure works can be illustrated by just one of the mediators which is released by the mast cell: histamine. (This name is already familiar if we have taken 'anti-histamine' drugs to relieve hay fever.) When it is released into the air passages and their underlying tissues, it can:

- irritate the nerves that control the smooth muscle surrounding

* IgE (Immunoglobulin Type E) is the chemical name for the antibodies.

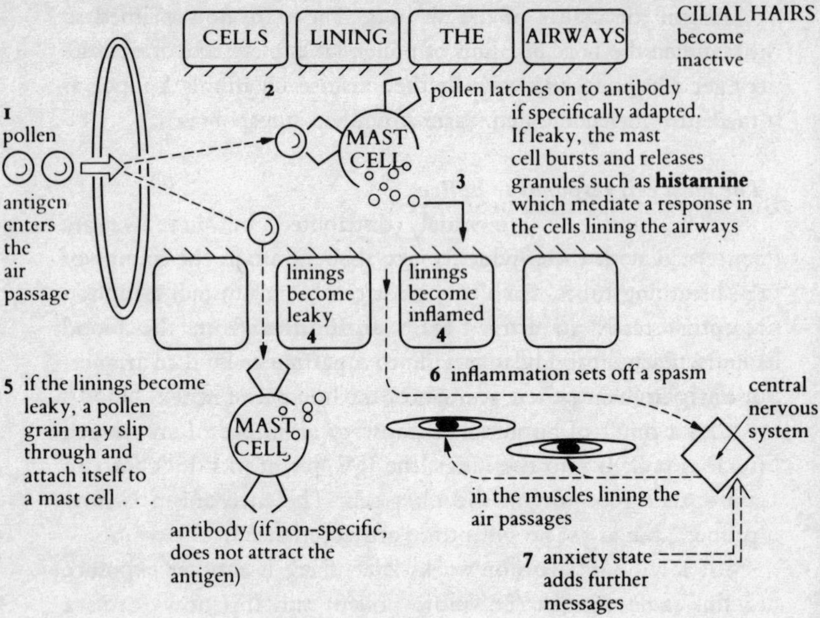

Fig. 5. A train of reactions

the breathing tubes so that the muscle thickens and narrows the airways

- make the mucus glands produce more mucus
- cause blood cells in the connective tissue to fill with blood and swell

This procedure is useful if it is attacking invaders, but not if, far from protecting our breathing, it goes over the top and impedes it.

We may recover naturally

With most allergic reactions of this kind the wheezing reaches a peak in about ten minutes. If there is no further invasion of the allergen (antigen), then the wheezing will decline in an hour or so and will disappear in a few hours more, even though no medicine has been taken. This response can be tested by measuring the calibre of the airways before, during and after a challenge by a single inhaled allergen, as described in Chapter Seven.

But the recovery may be delayed

In people who are allergic there may also be a delayed response which produces a more severe and persistent inflammation. It is not only histamine which is released from the mast cells but also leukotrienes and prostaglandins. These not only cause the smooth muscle to thicken, they also attract to the scene white blood cells, including eosinophils and neutrophils which have their origin in the bone marrow. These white blood cells carry antibodies on their surface and can in turn be switched on by the invading pollen. Neutrophils add to the swelling of the connective tissue. Eosinophils do even more damage because they can diminish the thin lining (epithelium) which protects the airways from invading irritants.

It is the arrival of these white blood cells which produces the delayed or second-phase response. This is more severe than the original attack of wheeziness; it may take hours, days or even weeks to disappear.

The molecular messengers

The process described above depends on an elaborate signalling system. This is carried out by messengers (or 'mediators').

This proceeds in the stages already described. At the first stage, messengers, such as histamine, convey signals to the airway muscles and cause them to contract. Contraction takes place when the calcium level inside each muscle cell rises, and this happens when histamine opens the gates to let in the calcium. The way the relieving drugs work is to shut the gates and to pump out the calcium. This activity is not affected by general calcium levels in the body.

The messengers which build the inflammatory process are called **cytokines**. They swim around in the fluids and have the ability to attract the inflammatory cells, make them active and take them to the site where the immune system requires them to operate. Chief among the cytokines are a varied family of **interleukins**.

It can be readily understood from this much-simplified account how an asthma attack builds and feeds on itself. The following diagram summarizes some of the activities involved in both inflammation and the contraction of airway muscles. The messengers are shown in *italics* and as ⟩⟩⟩ symbols:

	Allergen	**Mediator**	**Airway Muscles**
Stage one	mast cell or		
	macrophage ⟩⟩⟩	*histamine*	contract
	releases		
	cytokines		
	⟩⟩⟩		
Stage two:	inflammatory		
inflammation	cells summoned		
	⟩⟩⟩		
	epithelial	*(loss of mediator which*	
	lining attacked	*would relax the muscles)*	
	I		
	nerve endings		
	exposed ⟩⟩⟩	*acetylcholine*	contract
		neuropeptides	contract

The secret life of cells

By this stage the reader will have understood that the 'cells' involved in asthma are highly mobile, being carried in the bloodstream. I may not have conveyed the fact that they exist in vast numbers and can be counted in billions. This means that they are tiny and can be seen (with difficulty) only under powerful microscopes. 5,000 human cells would take up no more space than a grain of sand.

In spite of their minuscule size, each cell has a life of its own, taking in nourishment, which provides its own energy supply, and excreting its waste. At the heart of most cells is a nucleus, a command centre which regulates its activities. It also contains the chromosomes, the building bricks which form the DNA molecule.

Cells are born (many in the bone marrow), live and die. We have seen that they can send signals to other cells. In the airways they are of two kinds: there are the cells which arise within the airways (such as the lining cells), and there are the cells which arrive from outside, carried by the blood vessels, such as the lymphocytes and eosinophils.

Many of the white cells are 'phagocytic', that is they can gobble up other cells indiscriminately. They can break down to produce enzymes, which can also damage the airway tissues.

The cell that acts as a policeman

In the airways, as in other parts of the body, the **lymphocytes** are the recognition cells. They float around in the bloodstream and, when they meet another body, can instantly decide that it is foreign to them and then send a signal to the greedy scavenger (phagocytic) cells to deal with the intruder. They are like policemen on the beat calling for armed troops to restore order. This reaction is beneficial when there is damage to body-tissue. It is very undesirable when it takes it place in the breathing tubes and leads to asthma: the policeman becomes the chief criminal.

In people with asthma, the lymphocyte is likely to go into action when it meets any kind of antigen, be it an allergen or a virus. It responds by secreting both antibodies and its own messengers, known as lymphokynes, whose task is to summon the other white blood cells to the scene. This is the response which is described as inflammatory; for example, when the eosinophils arrive they constrict the airways both by increasing the discharge of mucus, causing the airway muscles to thicken, and by damaging the linings of the airways. This makes the airways much more responsive to a wider range of irritants, including histamine released from the mast cells. It explains why a breakdown of the mast cells, which in normal people would not cause asthma, in people with asthma irritates the airways sufficiently to do so. It is the lymphocytes which make the airways 'twitchy'.

This explanation also helps us to understand why steroids are so effective in preventing asthma: there is a great deal of evidence that steroids can prevent lymphocytes from becoming active. It also explains why inhaled steroids have to be taken on a daily basis to prevent asthma; the lymphocytes are always present in the bloodstream, ready to make their response to the antigens. Finally, it explains why it is so difficult to find a cure for asthma: it is the body's defence mechanism which is ultimately responsible for the attacks.

The scientists' task is made all the harder because all parts of the mechanism can influence one another through the system's very complicated circuitry. This means that, even though a scientist succeeds in blocking one pathway with the appropriate drug, another route is available by which the circuit can be switched on. It explains why drugs such as steroids, which intervene at an early stage in the cycle, are so valuable. Some of the pathways involved in the building of an asthma attack are shown diagrammatically in Figure 6, 'The full allergic response'.

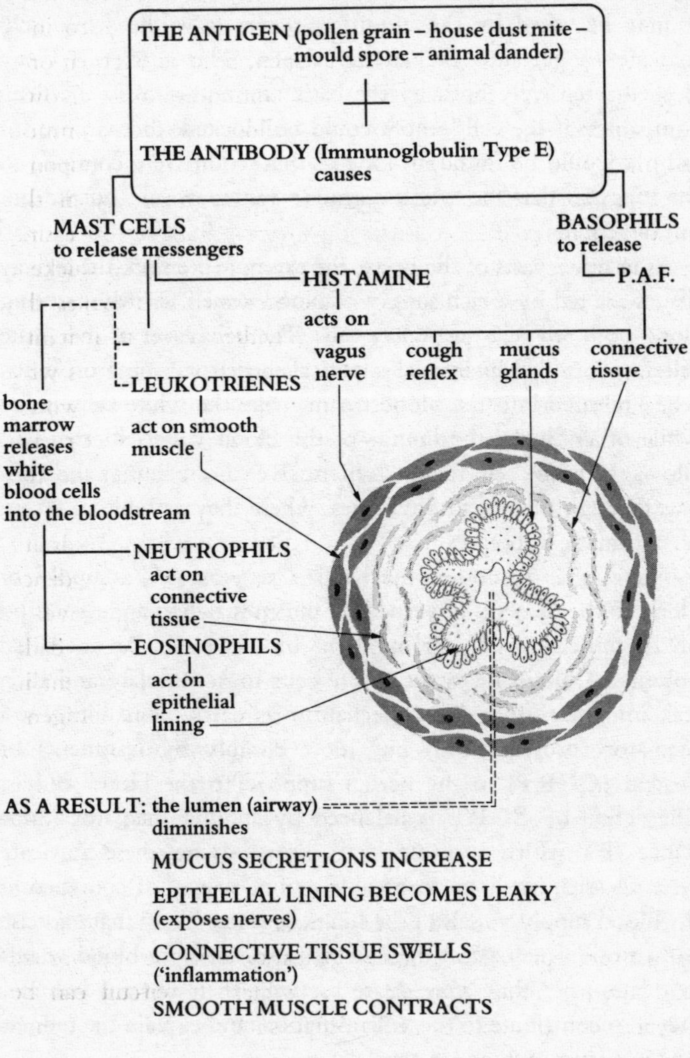

Fig. 6. Full allergic response (inflammation and secretion, as well as muscle spasm)

The role of the blood vessels

It may be asked by the inquiring reader how the white cells manage to get into the airway tissues. This matter is being studied intensively both by the basic scientists and by the drug companies: if the cells' entry could be blocked, then a cure for asthma would be found, as long as this action were confined to the lungs so that the whole immune system would not be put out of action.

As in other parts of the body, for example the skin, the airway tissues are fed by a rich supply of blood vessels, swiftly carrying along both red cells and white cells. The behaviour of the white cells is controlled by special chemical mediators, some of which when released into the bloodstream make the white cells sticky while others make the linings of the blood vessels sticky. This allows the white cells to attach themselves to the linings and then pass through them into the tissues, where they are able to set up the asthmatic response.

There is also another mechanism at work. The supply of blood to the tissues is governed by the constriction and dilatation of the muscles which surround the blood vessels. An increased volume of blood helps the white cells to accumulate and then leak into the tissues. This mechanism is partly controlled by a mediator (prostaglandin) but most durably by fragments of protein (CGRP) in the nerves supplied to the blood vessels. The action of CGRP is balanced by another mediator (Substance 'P') which can block it. By studying these intricate systems, scientists hope to be able to find a way of constricting the blood supply vessels in the lungs. It seems likely that exercise and emotion may affect these nerves and cause the blood vessels to dilate; since they may dilate to twice their normal volume, they also contribute to the 'inflammation' and explain the redness seen in airways which are constricted.

Irritable airways

So far we have concentrated on allergic asthma, brought about by inhaling pollen, dust mite droppings, moulds or animal dander. There are also non-allergic triggers which can affect anyone who has asthma. Examples are exercise and breathing cold and dry air, and inhaling fumes or smoke. These can lead to a spasm in the airway muscles, with little or no inflammation. When the challenge is removed, the airways recover and there is no increase in the underlying asthma.

The spasm is due to a nervous reflex like the reaction which takes place when a crumb enters the larger airways by mistake; in that case the crumb is forcibly expelled through a contraction of the chest muscles. In the smaller airways, when an irritant enters, the reflex causes the airway muscle to contract.

It is not certain why this happens, since the airway mucus is available to remove the irritant. It may be that in people with asthma the airways are leaky so that irritants reach the nerve endings. It is also likely that the mast cells can respond to irritants as well as to allergens, and release histamine. It is certain that the amount of water in the air we breathe is critical. If we breathe a dry vapour which has a higher than usual concentration of salts, this acts as an irritant, possibly because the airways lose water from their protective mucus blanket in order to replenish it. Cold fresh air irritates because it is drier than warm air.

The likelihood that irritants will cause spasm will increase if there is a virus infection, because this can damage the delicate protective lining of the air passages, allowing irritants to reach the mast cells and local nerve-endings.

Reversible and non-reversible asthma

The end result of these complex processes is **airway obstruction**. This refers to all the ways in which the **lumen** (inner space) of the air passages can be made smaller:

- o thickening and contraction of the smooth muscle which is wrapped round the airways
- o inflammation of the connective tissue
- o greatly increased secretion of mucus into the airways

In many people these responses are self-limiting or are easily reversed by the medicines. However, where the breathing tubes have become '**hyper-responsive**' (twitchy) on a permanent basis, the symptoms are likely to appear again in response to quite small challenges.

If the asthma has been both severe and persistent over many years, then the asthma may not be fully reversible because **scar tissue** is laid down in some of the airways and they become less 'elastic'. To this extent asthma can become non-reversible. Nowadays this process can usually be avoided if asthma is well controlled in the early years.

'Twitchy airways'

In the past, doctors thought that spasm of the airway muscles was the main cause of asthma; their efforts were concentrated on reversing it with bronchodilators. In the 1960s it became clear that inflammation is also present in some degree. Later research has shown how the two may be linked. This gave rise to the concept of 'twitchy airways' or **bronchial hyper-responsiveness** (B.H.R.). This can be illustrated with a simple diagram. An asthma attack will take place if

the airways are not very responsive or inflamed	*. . . but . . .*	**there is a very large trigger**
The airways are very responsive or inflamed	*. . . and . . .*	**there is quite a small trigger**

In non-asthmatic people, a trigger has to be very powerful and overwhelming to produce any narrowing in the airways – for example, a room full of dense smoke. In mild asthma, with airways either not at all or only slightly inflamed, it takes a sizeable trigger such as a heavy cold or a high pollen count or strenuous exercise to produce the symptoms of asthma. In people whose airways are more inflamed and 'hyper-responsive', it takes only a small trigger to cause the airway muscles to respond. In severe asthma we may find, for example, that moving from a warm room to a cooler one can cause breathlessness.

Two related conditions

The air sacs (alveoli) are where the gases are exchanged (oxygen taken in and carbon dioxide expelled). They are normally very elastic and inflate when air is breathed in. In **emphysema** this elasticity is diminished or destroyed, the lungs are over-expanded and enlarged. The supply of oxygen into the bloodstream is lessened, with a consequent loss of energy. Additional oxygen is supplied by tube from an oxygen cylinder or oxygen concentrator. Some people are born with a tendency to have emphysema; in others it is caused by air pollution due to smoking or working conditions. It may also be increased if scar tissue has formed in the airways as a result of prolonged and severe asthma.

In **bronchiectasis** the walls of the airways are damaged and the airways dilated. Removal of mucus is impaired and it can become infected. It may increase the asthmatic response to triggers and the inflammation caused by asthma. Treatment is through postural drainage and antibiotics.

Inheriting the allergy gene

People with asthma (or, for that matter, hay fever, eczema or urticaria), having read so far, will complain that I have not answered the question posed by the chapter title. They will ask: 'Why do I get it and not my neighbour . . . surely it must be inherited?' I asked a geneticist, Dr Bonnie Sibbald, to answer this question and what follows is based mainly on her fascinating reply.

It has long been known that allergic disorders have a genetic basis. This means that the genes we inherit from our parents through the union of eggs and sperm determine whether or not we will be susceptible to asthma or allergy. The evidence comes from the observation that asthma runs in families. However, this could be due to a shared environment rather than a shared inheritance of genes. So studies were conducted among twins. There is a closer resemblance in allergic responses among identical twins than among non-identical twins, and this demonstrates conclusively that a susceptibility to allergy (including asthma and hay fever) is inherited. Furthermore, in an as yet unborn baby with 'atopic' parents (i.e. subject to allergies), higher levels of an antibody (IgE) which contributes to allergic reactions can be detected in the blood in the umbilical cord than in 'normal' babies.

So the search began to track down which gene, along the winding string of DNA which is present in every cell, is responsible. A recent breakthrough has been achieved by researchers in Oxford. The method used is known as 'linkage analysis'. This is based on the principle that two genes which lie closely together on a single chromosome are less likely to become separated in the production of eggs or sperm than are genes which are widely separated or which are on two different chromosomes.

The scientists began to look for a 'marker gene'. This is a gene which is already well documented, in a huge library of such genes. They know where it is to be found on the DNA. They discover a large extended family (with four generations still living) which has lots of members with asthma. They select a marker gene and find out which variant of this gene is present in each member of the family. They then seek to discover if the people with allergy in the family all carry the same variant. If the answer is 'yes', then it must be that the marker gene lies close to the allergy gene on the chromosome.

This sounds straightforward until you realize that in the library there are millions of tiny genes in each cell and thousands of marker genes from which to choose. Dr Julian Hopkin and his colleagues at Oxford were lucky. They stumbled quite soon on a suitable marker gene and this showed that the allergy gene is somewhere on the short arm of chromosome 11. Their next task is to find out just where the gene is located along this arm.

It is likely to be many years before this results in a treatment which will succeed in blocking this gene. It must also be remembered that (unlike cystic fibrosis, which is wholly genetic) asthma and the other allergic illnesses are due both to a genetic inheritance and to triggers in the environment. It needs a powerful initial trigger to bring out the asthma, which explains why it skips some members of an atopic family, who remain free from allergy. As we shall see in Chapter Three, asthma may exist in people who are not allergic, and this too remains to be explained.

We are not yet in a position to breed asthma out of the population. We can, however, practise some sensible precautions. These are described in the next chapter. It is highly desirable, in the first six months of an infant's life, that all the indoor triggers should be reduced as far as possible; this will lessen the risk of the child becoming sensitized to them. This observation derives from research in Sweden, where it has been shown that it is those babies who are born in the short, three-week birch-pollen season who are most likely to develop an allergy to birch pollen. Research is under way that is confirming that this is true of all allergens when airborne (see page 46).

CHAPTER THREE

The Invisible Triggers

Reducing exposure to triggers

If you have managed to get through the previous chapter, you will be in no doubt that asthma is a complex illness which leads its sufferers to respond to very diverse triggers. Some of these are invisible and float in the air we all breathe; others arise from our lifestyle (what we do or eat, or from our work). Infection also puts asthmatics at risk.

triggers which are:	***triggers which are:***
'specific'	**'non-specific'**
'atopic'	**'non-allergic'**
'allergic'	**'irritants'**
seasonal	***all year round***
pollens	**exercise**
moulds	**emotions**
	atmosphere
all year round	**pollution**
house dust mite	**chemicals**
animals	**food additives**
certain foods	**infection**

triggers which can lead to the asthmatic response of airway obstruction

If you suffer from asthma mainly in the late spring and early summer, then it is probably due to an allergy to pollens. If the asthma persists into the autumn, then moulds are likely to be the triggers. If you have asthma all the year round, then it may be due additionally to an allergy to house dust mite, or to animals, or to food. On the other hand the trigger may be an irritant, such as a virus infection or air pollution. In this case the asthma is not due to allergy and can take place at all seasons.

There are three ways in which people with asthma (or hay fever) can try to prevent their attacks:

- they can try to reduce exposure to the triggers
- they can be 'de-sensitized'
- they can take appropriate medicines

In this chapter we will look at the triggers which provoke *asthma* and ask about each: 'Is there any way in which we can possibly avoid them?' We will also take a brief look at de-sensitization. *Hay fever* will be covered as a separate topic in Chapter Twelve, though the triggers are broadly the same as for asthma.

Pollens, moulds and dust

The flowers that bloom . . .

. . . do so in order to attract insects to the pollen. The pollen grains they produce do not travel very far, even in the spring and summer breezes, unless carried by insects. Cultivated flowers are not the main cause of pollen asthma, unless they are brought into the house. It is the lighter pollen grains from *wind-pollinated* plants (from trees, meadow grasses and weeds) that are mainly responsible for pollen asthma in those who are sensitive to it. In due season they produce pollen in clouds which can be carried by the wind for hundreds of miles.

In the United Kingdom the airborne pollen season lasts from March to September but reaches its peak with the grasses in June and early July. Leafy trees pollinate in the spring, like the birch from early April to mid-May; the London plane from early to late May. Grasses such as rye grass pollinate from late May to mid-August; wild flowers such as docks and nettles from June to late September. In Scotland this all happens a week or two later. Oil-seed rape is pollinated by insects (which upsets bee keepers) but the flowers release many volatile scents in May, and these can produce an allergic response at a distance.

Each country has its own special seasons for pollen allergy. In some parts of North America, for example, ragweed is a powerful source of wheezes, from August to September, and a single plant can release a million pollen grains in a day.

The local media publish average pollen counts. But these may conceal very high concentrations at certain times of the day, especially from 5 p.m. onwards. In fair weather, with a light and steady wind, pollens rise into the sky, high up in the clouds, during the morning. They descend again in the early evening. So it may be a good plan, during the pollen season, to open the windows only during the middle of the day. I have double-glazed the windows of my bedroom as an added precaution, and I close them after 4 p.m. Well-fitting outside doors are also advisable.

Though pollen is released most plentifully on sunny days, it is more likely to cause asthma in damp weather. Pollen grains are too large to penetrate the smaller airways but contain tiny particles (proteins) which are released in the moist air and are able to trigger asthma even in the tiniest airways. In fine weather the pollens are more likely to cause hay fever, because the whole grains land on the moist linings inside the nose and then open.

The best time to visit your garden is immediately after a heavy shower has washed all the pollen (but not the mould spores) out of the sky, and for just three to four hours afterwards.

The low allergen garden

Recently, a 'Low Allergen Garden' was created for the National Asthma Campaign at the Chelsea Flower Show, the first of its kind. Apart from banishing most wind-pollinated plants, we also excluded two families of flowers which are especially likely to cause allergy: the daisy family (*compositae*) of asters, chrysanthemums and dahlias; and the *pinks* (including carnations). Heavily scented flowers and shrubs were avoided, because scent may itself be a trigger, but this still left a huge range of plants from which to choose.

In the Low Allergen Garden there is no grass, because mowing causes real difficulties; grass collects dust and pollens in large amounts. Instead there are terraces. Weeding is kept down by mulches such as gravel which will not encourage moulds (see below) and by ground cover plants. Gravel does not supply humus so it needs a rich soil underneath, at least two feet of it if fruit trees are to be grown. There are no hedges, because these gather dust and pollen from elsewhere, but trelliswork with climbers is used instead.

Fruit trees are allowed, because they are insect-pollinated; a herb garden can be included with the advice that the herbs should be cut before flowering; if dried, they should be kept in an outbuilding. Low-scented roses are acceptable, in the garden at least.

Other measures

Is there anything else you can do to escape a trigger such as pollen which is everywhere in the atmosphere?

- Offices with efficient air-conditioning keep out pollens.

- In the country, the car (with all the windows shut) can be a temporary refuge from pollen, to help bring an attack of hay fever or asthma under control.

○ It has been suggested that you rinse your hair to rid it of pollen before you retire; dogs, which bring in pollen on their fur, should ideally be kept outside during the peak season.

○ Choosing a suitable place for a holiday, to escape from pollens at home, is not all that easy. There is a problem of timing, because our season can vary by a couple of weeks, delayed by a cool spring. It is a good plan to choose somewhere in the mountains or close to offshore breezes. A sea breeze in the afternoon is usually free from pollen but the breezes reverse in the evening. (See also Chapter Nine.)

Dust that builds on dust

One of the more imaginative English eccentrics, Mr Quentin Crisp, who used to be a familiar figure in Chelsea, has pointed out that if you leave dust well alone it never rises above a certain thickness; much better not to disturb it. Unfortunately this does not work, because we stir it all the time.

The dust particles that trigger attacks of asthma have to be small enough to penetrate the smallest breathing tubes; to be 'allergic' they have to be derived from living matter.

What is dust? We tend to think of it as something that comes in from outside. This is only a small part of the story! Pollens from grasses and weeds can be transferred from outside into the house, for example by animals. Arising from within, there are the skin scales shed by humans and pets; there are fragments of clothing and bedding and debris from upholstery; dust from the fireplace, from dead insects, dead plant matter; food fragments, tobacco shreds and, above all, the house dust mite.

The house dust mite

The allergen that features at the top of our hit list, in that up to three-quarters of patients with asthma are sensitive to it, is

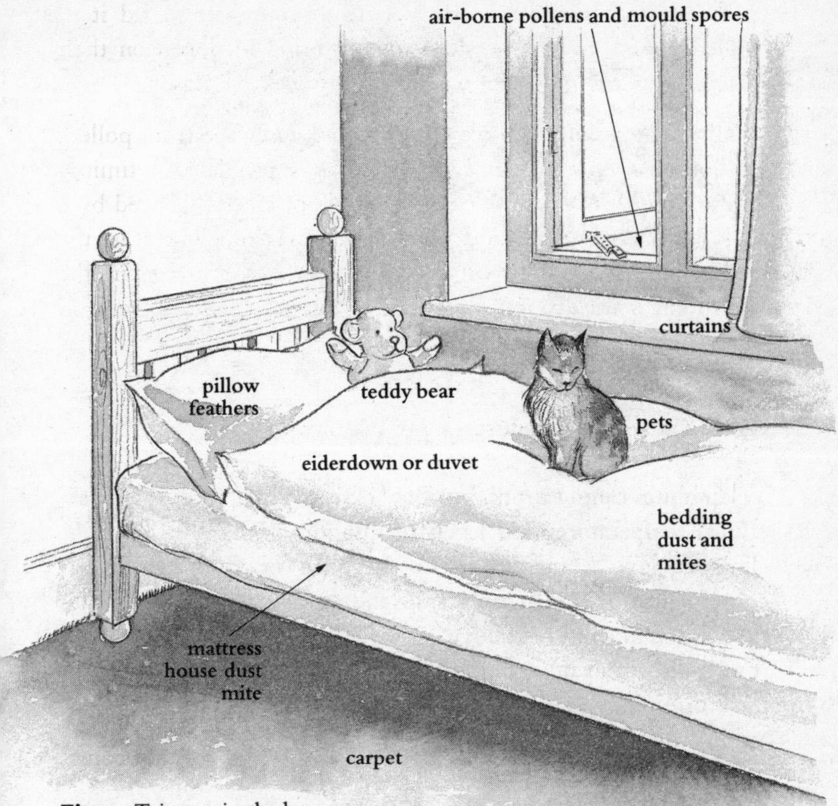

Fig. 7. Triggers in the home

produced by the **house dust mite**. This animal is 0.3 mm long and is invisible to the naked eye, even in large numbers. In its common form it is called rather grandly *Dermatophagoides pteronyssimus*; it is blind and, suitably enlarged, could play a leading role in a horror movie. It starts as an egg, becomes a six-legged larva, emerges as an eight-legged mite and especially likes to live in mattresses (where it is present in millions), duvets, feather pillows, thick carpets and soft toys. The mites feed on shed skin scales (human and animal, including feathers and wool) and on any moulds which may also be present.

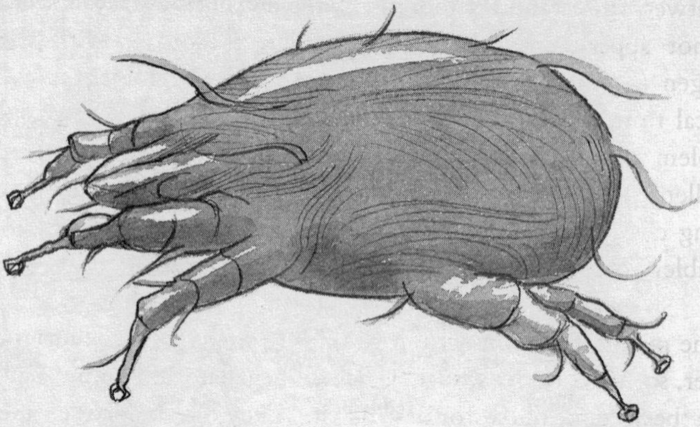

Fig. 8. The house dust mite

The mites cannot drink, but they extract water from the air at critical temperatures and levels of humidity. Reproduction declines at low temperatures, so they can be frustrated by a combination of low temperature and low humidity. They are killed at temperatures above 55°C (which is not tolerated by most pillow and quilt fillings). Even if the mites are removed, their droppings may remain and be in a potent state to cause asthma.

It is not the mite itself which enters our airways but fragments of its faecal pellets, light enough to become and to remain airborne, and small enough to enter the smallest airways. The allergen involved is an enzyme which is labelled Der-p-1. It is likely to be distributed all around the house. Studies in Poole, U.K., suggest an alarming increase, in recent years, in the sensitivity of children to Der-p-1. There are many similar mites which can cause asthma, for example grain storage mites.

War on the house dust mite

There is growing evidence that people first become 'sensitized' to house dust mite allergen (Der-p-1) in early infancy, especially at between three and six months of age, even though symptoms do not appear until the child is older. If contact with this allergen (and other domestic allergens) can be avoided at this critical time, there is a good chance that it will not be a major problem in later years. At any age it is sensible to reduce the load of allergens, especially in the bedroom and (where there are young children) in the living room as well. What measures are possible? Sources of equipment are given on page 285.

○ The mite is not an insect but belongs to the same family as the spider, so ACARICIDES, such as benzyl benzoate and tannic acid, have been developed to destroy it. They are effective, but repeated applications are needed and they should not be used on pillows or mattresses except as a preliminary to stringent cleaning routines and encasing with special barrier textiles. They do not remove the accumulated allergens, so intensive vacuum-cleaning (mattress or carpet) or hot washing (pillows and duvets) is needed afterwards. See 'Allersearch', page 285.

○ Our grandparents lived in homes which were WELL VENTILATED. Our softer generation tries to live in a Mediterranean climate. When we install double glazing, we raise the humidity to a point at which mites can thrive. This is because humans give off moisture, which remains in the room. Mites thrive best at around 75 per cent relative humidity; they do not breed at under 50 per cent humidity. But people who install de-humidifiers have to be careful not to dry the air too much.

○ Houses at Aarhus in Denmark have been designed specially for people with asthma. Using double glazing, they incorporate a system whereby incoming air is filtered, de-humidified and also warmed by the extracted air (see page 57).

○ FREE-STANDING AIR FILTERS have been aggressively promoted by high-pressure sales methods not unlike pyramid selling. The salesmen's claims should be treated with caution, if only because airborne allergens are constantly replenished and it would take a whirlwind to remove them! There is, as yet, no evidence that electrostatic filtering systems are beneficial, but 'HEPA' (high efficiency particulate air) filters may help reduce symptoms if other methods of control have been used as well.

○ VACUUM-CLEANING has been mentioned. Unfortunately, mites cling to the fabric with suckers on their feet, and in any case some eggs are likely to remain to start a new generation. Most domestic dry vacuum-cleaners leak fine particles through the bag and they remain suspended for a time. Clean every day in a dull light when the mites are likely to be closer to the surface, and ventilate the room afterwards. Always discard the bag immediately after cleaning, or the mites will crawl back again! The ideal cleaner must have adequate power to provide good suction, plus a double-thickness dust bag and a system of exhaust microfilters to prevent the vacuumed dust from being returned to the air.

○ MEDICAL DRY VACUUM-CLEANERS trap all but the smallest particles but they are expensive, and it has not been established beyond doubt whether they are all effective. Clean every day for the first seven days, then regularly every week. Models are available from Medivac (Microfilter MO2), ALT (Compact Electronic 406), DeLuxe (607), Miele and, for 100% efficiency, Vorwerk.

○ WET VACUUM CLEANING has been shown to increase mite populations unless solvents and wetting agents are used (the 'Vax' method can reduce mite populations in carpets and mattresses).

○ Always use a slightly DAMP DUSTER, to avoid spreading the dust. Clean under the bed and on top of the door frames, pictures and mouldings, as well as the more obvious places. Avoid upholstered furniture in the bedroom, and heavy curtains or venetian blinds. Roller blinds with a plastic finish are best. Wash light curtains regularly. Keep ornaments in glass cabinets.

o A HOT WASH (above 55°C) will kill mites in soft furnishings, soft toys and bedding. Duvets collect the greatest amount of mites, so they need the same treatment. Sheets should be ironed.

o It is preferable that carpets, blankets and duvets, in fact all soft furnishings, should be made from ARTIFICIAL FIBRES. As explained, they provide less food for the mites and also carry a higher electrostatic charge than natural fibres; this holds in some of the dust. The ideal room would not have carpets but sealed flooring or linoleum, or polished wooden floors. Rugs can be exposed to sunlight and beaten, but should not be shaken in the home.

o Clothes left scattered in the bedroom will be quickly colonized by mites. They should be kept in drawers or closed wardrobes.

o In 1547 John Hamilton, the Archbishop of St Andrews in Scotland, was visited by a famous physician, astrologer and philosopher, Geronimo Cardano of Pavia. On learning that His Grace had severe asthma, the visitor recommended that the feather pillows be replaced by wooden ones. Nowadays we use pillows and quilts filled with terylene. This is an improvement, but they should withstand a wash above 55°C (check the label before purchase).

o A large reduction of mites in mattresses and carpets can be achieved by a combination of a freezing agent (LIQUID NITROGEN) and thorough vacuum-cleaning afterwards. Soft toys which collect dust should be frozen, or washed each week in very hot water. Few mites survive at temperatures below 5°C.

o A mattress may contain millions of mites, soon replenished if a few eggs remain after cleaning. One allergist has suggested that the population can be diminished by using an ELECTRIC BLANKET to lower the humidity. This will not change the amount of allergenic dust. Avoid a padded headboard – a perfect home for mites!

o The experts give a qualified approval to the measures

mentioned above. They are currently much more enthusiastic about the use of specially treated ALLERGEN EXCLUSION BARRIERS to enclose pillows and mattresses. These have two aims: to provide a complete barrier against mite allergen and to allow water vapour (which we generate) to pass through. They have to be 'breathable'. They are at the same time waterproof.

This can be achieved in two ways. 'Microporous' fabrics have a plastic layer or membrane which lets through the water-vapour molecules by way of tiny pores in the plastic. More recently, a polyurethane fabric has been introduced. This is permeable to water vapour because the plastic layer is very thin and it also has an affinity for water molecules. The most recent fabric ('Alprotec') is less expensive than its predecessors and even less resistant to water vapour. Slumberland produce a Health Seal range.

The water-vapour-permeable covers are used next to the mattress, duvet or pillow and are covered with the usual decorated cotton or terylene outer covers. They are wiped down with a damp cloth when the sheets are changed and washed when needed or dry cleaned, and then aired.

If you cannot afford a barrier cover, then *two* layers of sheets, duvet covers or pillow cases will afford some protection.

o We could leave our present homes and go and live in the high MOUNTAINS. Above 2,000 metres, the air is so dry that neither the mites nor the moulds on which they partly feed can survive. This explains why allergic people often feel better after a holiday in the Alps, if only for a short while. They soon become re-sensitized when they return home.

Anti-mite measures: a summary

Much work remains to be done by zoologists and allergists to discover really efficient and safe ways of frustrating house dust mites. A Working Group which met in Southampton, in Southern England, in 1991 concluded that no single method will suffice. It must be emphasized that the mites are everywhere in the home, at all times of the year.

Intensive and regular vacuum-cleaning, together with textiles and pillows made from synthetic fibres, the treatment of old mattresses with an acaracide or liquid nitrogen before they are vacuum-cleaned and then encased inside a water-vapour-permeable or microporous cover; and plenty of fresh air to reduce the humidity . . . if all these measures are combined, then significant reductions in mite populations will be achieved. When young children are involved, not only the bedroom but also the living room should be attacked in this way. Air filters can be added, but they will be of little use by themselves.

Inflammation due to allergy may persist for some weeks, so do not look for instant improvement in symptoms, but a gradual reduction.

Domestic pets and other animals

Allergists are severe about pets. They tell us that any animal, large or small, can sensitize an atopic (potentially allergic) person and be the first cause of a child becoming asthmatic. This danger may not be evident for some time, unless a skin prick test is carried out, and these are seldom used nowadays. This kind of allergy may be compared to a time bomb ticking away unnoticed. At first the symptoms are suppressed with medicines, but the sensitivity only increases, so more powerful treatments are needed. It would be far better to put the family's health at the forefront and find a good home for the pet elsewhere, perhaps to be visited occasionally. It is rare for a child or an adult to be sensitive only to animals. However, this is not an argument for keeping them, since one allergy reinforces another. Remove one and you may reduce the impact of the rest.

Only a brief exposure is needed to cause symptoms which may persist, for example a necessary visit to a relative who keeps cats. Animals can cause sensitivity even though there is no direct contact. Dr Morrow Brown has cited the example of a mother who suddenly developed asthma because her daughter took up riding and threw her contaminated clothes into the family washing basket. When buying a house, try to make sure that the previous owners did not keep any pets.

Raining cat and dog allergen

About 40 per cent of children with asthma are 'sensitized' to cats and/or dogs. When a cat or dog is first introduced, the allergens are soon distributed around the home and hide away in nooks and crannies to become airborne when disturbed. If the animal is removed, the allergens may remain for months in the furnishings unless rigorous cleaning is undertaken.

The main cat allergen is labelled Fel-d-1 and is found in the saliva and sebum which coat the fur during grooming and which become volatile, airborne in very small particles that are easily inhaled. This explains why someone who is allergic to cats can react when entering a room, even though the cat is absent. Some breeds are thought to be especially potent sources of cat allergen (Siamese and Burmese). In extremely suggestible persons who have been conditioned by the response from a real cat, just the picture of a cat may be enough to start a wheeze.

While cats lick themselves, dogs are keen on licking any human whom they regard as an acceptable pack-leader, including children. This can cause not only asthma but also urticaria, a skin rash. Dander (dandruff), saliva and hair are sources of the allergen Can-f-1, and it is found in many breeds with both short and long hairs. As in cats, sensitization is most likely in the first year of a child's life.

A skin test would confirm whether a dog, cat, horse or other animal is responsible for the asthma. The tests are carried out in just a few large teaching hospitals and are not always reliable, as explained on page 55; they should be highly specific. If the saliva, of, say, a male Siamese is what is suspected, this is what should be used, in solution, in the test, if available.

Replacing the pet dog or cat with a rabbit, gerbil, guinea pig or hamster is not a good idea. These animals are used by laboratory workers and a high proportion of technicians develop asthma as a result. This is partly caused by the urine, which becomes volatile and gives off its characteristic smell. It can take eighteen months for a child to be sensitized by them. Even tropical fish, which look much too beautiful to harm anyone, may cause their owner to become sensitized – not to the fish themselves but to their food, such as ants' eggs. It seems that many Russians, who like to keep tropical fish in their apartments, suffer in this way.

Insects can be dangerous

It is well known that insects can cause allergic reactions through their stings, sometimes with severe consequences. The area round the sting may remain swollen for a day: this need be no cause for alarm unless the swelling persists or the whole arm or leg swells. In that case you should see a doctor at once because you may be suffering from 'anaphylactic shock'. This is like a very severe asthma attack and may lead to loss of consciousness and even death. Incidentally, it is the saliva of a mosquito which causes an allergic reaction, injected along with the sting.

A mouldy business

If you feel wheezy when you stand near a stack of rotting compost or when passing fields freshly turned over by the plough or in a damp basement, then you are probably allergic to moulds. If you feel better when the landscape is covered with snow, then this confirms it. About 5 per cent of people with asthma are sensitive to moulds.

Mould spores come from fungi, which live on rotting vegetation and in damp housing. They produce pollen-like spores which become airborne in their millions. Moulds tend to lie dormant during the cold months, wake into life in the spring and remain active until well into the autumn. Very high levels are reached when the air is damp, especially at night.

Moulds like warm damp places, such as grass-clippings and forests. The rich warm smell of newly ploughed fields comes from moulds. I moved to the seaward side of the New Forest in the hope of escaping from pollens but the asthma subsequently became worse. I read that in the Middle Ages the monks in nearby Beaulieu Abbey suffered badly from asthma – this may have been the forest moulds, as well as the oak-tree pollens. Ripe crops of wheat, oats and barley produce moulds.

Common moulds in summer include *Cladosporium* and *Alternaria*, which are found both indoors and outside. Inside the home, mildew (*Penicillium*) and *Cladosporium* can thrive on damp wallpaper and old clothes. *Aspergillus*, which causes a severe form of asthma, likes rotting vegetation.

Inside the home, moulds flourish not only in damp basements, on old wallpaper and upholstery, but even in modern foam furniture and rubber pillows when damp. Clothes in a badly ventilated wardrobe can grow moulds. So can vegetable bins, pet litter and potted plants. If allergic to moulds, you may be brave enough to remove the wallpaper and use emulsion paint instead. You should get rid of all the rejected odds and ends which lie around in corners. It is impossible to treat upholstery with any success, and foam filling should be replaced from time to time. Clothes should be dry-cleaned regularly. Sheets, duvets and blankets should be aired outside, but not in the pollen season. The bathroom carpet should be replaced with vinyl or linoleum.

Double glazing helps to increase moulds. The air inside the house, when the windows are shut, can be kept moving with electric fans. But this means that the floors should be kept free from dust: fans push it up into the breathing tubes.

Some modern office ventilating systems grow moulds in the ducts and then spread them over the inmates, along with bacteria, viruses, pollen and air pollutants. It is not easy to escape from moulds.

One man's meat is another man's poison

This is as true today as it was when first observed, in Roman times. Allergy to food receives a lot of attention nowadays, but chest physicians do not see it as a common cause of asthma. They also doubt whether avoiding action is sensible, except in those patients where the allergy can be traced to one particular type of food which can be eliminated and still leave the patient with a balanced diet. They take the view that it is simpler to rely on the medicines – especially since these have to be taken anyway, as asthma usually has many other triggers in addition to food.

That having been said, allergists are concerned that our complex factory-made foods may be contributing to the rising incidence of asthma, and they feel that serious attention should be paid to the substances added to ready-cooked foods. This topic will be discussed at greater length in Chapter Eleven.

How can I tell what causes my allergies?

We have already seen how allergic persons develop antibodies against allergens such as pollen grains or house dust. When the allergen and the antibody meet, chemicals such as histamine are released into the sensitive tissues.

If histamine is released into the nostrils and eyelids, you start sneezing and itching (hay fever); if it is released into the breathing tubes, you become wheezy (asthma). If, on the other hand, it is released into the skin, an itchy swelling appears. This reaction is quite small and harmless, so doctors use it to find out what substances you are allergic to – or, rather, they used to do so, because the tests are not widely used nowadays.

This technique is called a skin prick test. The doctor drops a small extract of allergen suspended in water on to the skin of your forearm and then scratches it into the skin. By testing a range of different allergens in this way he can discover whether you are allergic (atopic) to various pollens (tree and grass), animals, house dust mite extract or moulds. If a small, reddish, itchy swelling appears then you are allergic to the substance in the extract. The test has a few limitations:

o It is possible to be atopic (positive results from the test) without ever having any symptoms of asthma or hay fever.

o It is possible to be atopic but to develop asthma from a cause which is not allergic, as for example a chemical at work or the intake of cold air.

o Some people are atopic to one substance only: they are allergic only to cats or to certain foods such as shellfish. But most asthma sufferers are allergic to more than one substance, and many are atopic to all the extracts, though in varying degrees as between one extract and another. In these latter cases, avoiding the substances is difficult, even impossible, and reliance on medical treatment alone would seem to be preferable.

A skin test can have some advantages. It can help the doctor confirm that the wheeziness is indeed an asthmatic response and is not due to some other lung disorder. It can help support the patient's own belief that a particular substance is responsible, and confound those who doubt this. And it can be a guide to treatment, for example, by suggesting to a horse-loving girl that she should take her medicine before setting out for the stables.

Home sweet home

Having done our best to frustrate dust, animal dander, smokers and other triggers, we are still left with a nagging worry about the air we breathe inside our homes. What is the ideal temperature? And the ideal humidity?

To frustrate the house dust mite we need to open the windows wide and to switch off the central heating for long periods. But this will let in air which is full of pollen, or fumes, or is too cold for our sensitive airways, especially at night.

So we are left with the common-sense idea that we let in fresh air when we can, when the bedroom is not in use, but keep the night-time temperature at a level which our airways will tolerate, and we try to keep pollen out in the grass pollen season. We have to work out by trial and error what inside conditions suit us best and then try to persuade everyone else to adapt to them – not an easy task, since people have very firm views about the kind of atmosphere that suits them.

One of the reasons why we get more colds in winter is that we congregate together in airless rooms and exchange germs. On the other hand, the cold virus multiplies less by direct contact than as a result of falls in the temperature which lower our resistance to it.

The low-allergen house

In Denmark in the 1980s an unique experiment was started. At Aarhus, houses were designed and built specially for people with severe asthma. The aim was to reduce concentrations of house dust mites while maintaining a warm temperature. The mites cannot drink and they absorb water from the air, so low humidity is maintained. Moist air is extracted and its heat is used to warm filtered, dry, incoming air. This is vented into each room. There is double glazing throughout and an absence of carpets. The occupiers enjoy living in their homes and have reported a great improvement in their asthma, and the dust mite population is much lower than in a normal house (see page 286).

Asthma in warm, dry climates

Given that warm air suits sensitive airways better than cold air, and that dry air frustrates mites, it might be supposed that the incidence of asthma is lowest in the warmest and driest climates. This is not necessarily so. Wagga Wagga, in the dry wheat-growing belt of New South Wales, has the same prevalence of asthma as Sydney, which has a damp climate. Saudi Arabia was relatively free from asthma until heavily scented flowering shrubs were planted in Riyadh. And Tucson, in the Arizona desert, used to be a haven for people with asthma until they decided to fill it with beautiful trees and flowers!

Why de-sensitization is out of favour

De-sensitization is not used very much nowadays. Why is this? The simple answer is that the newer medicines enable physicians to control asthma much more successfully, so the process is no longer needed except where a life may be at risk from a particular substance such as a bee sting or exposure to a cat.

The aim is to change the allergic response by giving an allergen in a very small dose and then increasing it on a weekly basis until the patient can tolerate levels of the allergen that would normally cause asthma. The allergen is identified with skin prick tests. Treatment, which starts six months before the period which causes the trouble, is in the form of an extract which is injected under the skin of the arm. For year-round allergens a maintenance level is reached and the dose is repeated, at this level, every month.

De-sensitization is now confined to special centres. This is because there may, rarely, be a life-threatening response and the doctor has to have adrenaline on hand to counter this. The injected substance has to be highly specific, for example from the appropriate breed of cat. The procedure is expensive and time-consuming. The majority of chest physicians believe that a better degree of control can be achieved by using the preventive medicine, and by avoiding very specific allergens.

Non-allergic triggers: exercise, emotions and chemicals

Many report that in middle age and afterwards the non-allergic triggers become more noticeable and the allergens (pollens, mould spores, house dust) not quite so troublesome as before. This is a normal pattern. It occurs presumably because our immune reactions slow down when we grow older so that on the one hand we become more vulnerable to infections, and at the same time less liable to respond to allergens.

Asthma due to exercise

Most people with asthma find that, at times, exercise is a trigger. In the young this response can usually be prevented with the appropriate medicine; in older people with severe and persistent asthma, this becomes more difficult to achieve.

A curious feature of asthma induced by exercise is that it gets worse after the exercise has finished, reaching a peak after a few minutes and then lasting for about half an hour, before it subsides. What happens is that at first exercise dilates the airways. Needing more air when we exercise, we take in a greater volume; this, even in summer, is relatively cool and dry compared with the warm moist air needed for passage through into the air sacs. Faced with such a large volume, the nasal passages are not able to condition it; the breathing tubes have to complete this task, so they lose water and the protection of the moist mucus blanket. The airways become 'leaky', the nerves which lie under the linings are triggered and airway muscles contract.

Does this mean that we should give up taking exercise? The answer is an emphatic 'no', but we should adjust the exercise to what can be tolerated. There is no doubt that exercise taken in moderation can benefit everyone. It builds strong healthy children, provides a challenge for adolescents who are keen on sport, and in middle age helps keep heart disease at bay. In old age it helps avoid a tendency of muscles to sag. It helps fight infections and improves the efficiency of breathing so that we can perform better with fewer resources. Some doctors go further and claim that physically fit people are better able to cope with mental stress than those who are unfit; they have a sense of well-being, are more confident and meet challenges more easily.

Those of us who have asthma need to know how we can tolerate exercise. Some forms cause more wheeziness than others. It depends on how much lung power is needed. Running is worse than riding a horse or cycling. Swimming causes very little wheeziness: the body is supported and the warm moist atmosphere of a heated indoor pool is ideal for people with asthma (see page 191).

How do you decide whether you stand in need of more exercise? You take a watch with a second hand and go to the foot of the stairs. Step on the bottom stair with one foot; bring the other up to it and then step down. Repeat the exercise 24 times within 60 seconds and then stop. After a further 60 seconds, take your pulse rate for a period of 15 seconds. You should count no more than 25 heartbeats for men and 28 for women under the age of forty-five. If your rate is above 20, you are unfit and would benefit from exercise.

How much exercise is needed? If you work out twice a week for 20–30 minutes vigorously enough to increase the breathing rate, this should be sufficient. But, you may object, even this modest amount may induce an attack of wheezing. This is an understandable worry – but there are various ways in which exercise can be tolerated by people whose asthma is normally affected by it.

o You can take medicine beforehand, as explained on page 131. A peak flow meter will help decide whether the asthma is sufficiently controlled to undertake the exercise (explained on page 152).

○ Fitness can be acquired through a graduated swimming programme because of all exercises this is the least likely to provoke wheeze. The asthmatic can then progress to what we used to refer to at school as 'physical jerks' but which are now described less alarmingly as 'dry land' exercises. All the exercises should start gently with warming-up movements before becoming more strenuous. This enables the lungs to adapt gradually to the demands being imposed on them.

○ Many athletes, including some Olympic gold medallists, have asthma; they find that, before a long distance run, a few short sharp sprints will release enough natural adrenaline to keep the breathing tubes relaxed. If exercise makes you short of breath, then an energetic sprint on the spot may do the same trick and prevent subsequent activity from provoking asthma.

In cold weather I stay indoors and rely on a folding exercise bicycle. Physiotherapists tell me that this is an excellent way of keeping fit. Unlike ordinary cycling, you can read at the same time!

The role of the physiotherapist

Physiotherapists are usually attached to hospitals, but some health centres employ one. They are especially good at communicating the skills needed to control asthma, such as the proper use of inhalers. They can discuss the trigger factors and teach correct breathing and relaxation. They can also show how the asthmatic can be taught to tolerate exercise.

The habit of relaxation and relaxed breathing, learnt when free of an asthmatic attack, can be a great help in the earlier stages of an attack. Relaxation can be either general or local. By general relaxation the physiotherapist means letting go of each muscle one by one, starting with the toes and working up through the whole body, so that all tension slips away. You may ask whether this cannot be achieved in sleep. But we may sleep in a way that is tense and unrelaxed, and sleep does not remove all tension. Local relaxation is aimed at the shoulders and chest muscles and teaches you to check whether these are as relaxed as you suppose.

Some years ago I went to the Brompton Hospital in London to make a film for doctors about breathing exercises. The superintendent physiotherapist told me that I would be the first to benefit: 'You are a shallow breather,' she told me. I have read recently that I probably share this characteristic with most of the population: we simply fail to use our lungs properly, breathing only with the upper part of the lungs and leaving the old stale air in the lower part. In contrast dogs, cats and other non-human animals generally take full breaths every time, to their great advantage. 'Diaphragmatic breathing', which should be a normal way of breathing, is welcomed by mothers as something they can teach to their asthmatic child. It consists in learning to breathe gently from the bottom of the lungs.

What specialists do not endorse is the idea that we can be usefully trained to move one part of the chest independently of all the other parts. In practice, the accessory muscles (those between the ribs and, during exercise, around the neck and shoulders) are brought into play just as and when we need them.

In severe asthma there may be an excess of secretions in the lungs; a physiotherapist can teach 'postural drainage' to help clear this and make breathing easier. A lying position on a firm support, tilted to provide the drainage, is accompanied by one or two 'huffs' to help move the secretions from the lower to the upper air passages. This helps only when the asthma attack is over.

Over-breathing

This should not be confused with the faster breathing that is needed in an attack to provide sufficient oxygen when deeper breathing is not possible. Over-breathing means 'hyper-ventilation', or breathing at a greater rate than the body needs at the time. In asthmatics this panting is sometimes attributed to our understandable anxiety. It may simply mean being out of breath through exercise taken when we are unfit.

When the rate of breathing is increased in this way, there is no significant increase in the take-up of oxygen by the blood, but it can reduce the waste gas (carbon dioxide) to an excessive extent. This has many undesirable results because carbon dioxide is not simply a by-product of respiration, it is also a regulator of the central nervous system. If the pressure of carbon dioxide in the blood falls to a small extent, through just a moderate degree of over-breathing, this results in a speeding up of nervous impulses, an increase in sympathetic activity (the 'fight or flight' response) which dilates the breathing tubes, and hearing and sight become more acute. If, however, the carbon dioxide pressure falls to a severe extent, these reactions are reversed. This results in a slowing of brain function and an increase in parasympathetic activity. This leads not only to dizziness, headache, cramp, sweating and a feeling of anxiety but also to a constriction of the airways. If over-breathing continues for a few minutes, the automatic impulse to breathe is switched off and the patient turns blue. Occasionally children use this ruse to frighten their parents and get their own way.

The remedy for hyper-ventilation is to practise controlled breathing in the non-asthmatic state. In a very severe attack, however, voluntary control of the breathing rate may be impossible.

One consequence of over-breathing helps to explain how in tribal ceremonies the initiates are able to endure mutilation and other trials. The dancing, singing and excitement of the ceremony lead to hyper-ventilation and after a time this can decrease the sensation of pain.

Getting excited or upset

According to Sir John Floyer, writing in 1698, 'All Asthmatics, being angry or sad, do fall into fits oftener than when they are cheerful.' Some of us suspect that he may have been confusing the effect and the cause, or simply reporting his own experience.

That emotions can cause breathlessness will be accepted by anyone who has choked with laughter, become breathless with excitement or had to make a speech in public. In normal people such responses are short-lived, but in asthma-sensitive people they may be prolonged. This may be simply due to the extra volume of cool air which reaches the breathing tubes, or to over-breathing, or to an increase in the blood supply to the airways, carrying with it invading white cells.

Scientists have demonstrated, by showing a particularly frightening film to a group of asthmatics, that airway obstruction can increase even when the rate of breathing is unchanged. We might expect the opposite result, since the sympathetic system's 'fight or flight' response prepares the body for action by opening the airways, and adrenaline is released in response to stress. However, when anxiety is prolonged, it tends to constrict the airways. At times the illness feeds on itself, as when we find that we have left the inhaler behind when away from home. On the way back, when relief is in prospect, the wheezing may diminish. And when we are wholly absorbed in a creative pursuit we often forget about the wheezes altogether. We may even be affected by the colour of our walls: lavender, and green, are said to relax the airways!

Much has been written about the way emotions may reinforce an attack of asthma. Little has been said about the devastating way in which asthma can spoil relations with other people. This will be one of the topics reserved for Chapter Thirteen.

A musical interlude

At a local branch meeting of the National Asthma Campaign we had a talk from an opera singer who suffers from asthma, Mr Howard Milner. Many singers have asthma, or at any rate use relieving inhalers at critical times.

Singing is all about the even and controlled exhalation of air, and singers with asthma who work at their breath control can greatly improve their asthma. If preventive medicine is indicated, they prefer Intal or Tilade, since the inhaled steroids remove the upper harmonics from the sound.

Singing predates human speech and probably first existed through mothers crooning to their babies, then extended to the cries of hunters. These sounds served to express feelings directly and this is what every singer must learn to do.

We were invited to make those primal noises (Mmmmmmmmmm ... Nnnnnnnnn) and feel the breathing muscles working especially in the lower torso. This is in contrast to asthma, which makes you breathe in a shallow way. Relaxation helps as well, especially before a performance. All the muscles should work together, in harmony.

The exercises we then followed were not unlike those which used to be commonplace in asthma management. For the address of the Association for Voice Movement Therapy see Chapter Seventeen.

The mysterious effect of the atmosphere

Most normal people are aware that the weather can raise or depress their spirits; but asthmatics, with their super-sensitive airways, can react to quite small changes in weather conditions. Some are particularly upset by cold damp airstreams, others by hot dry weather. Summer thunderstorms make us reach for our inhalers, and so do autumn mists. In severe asthma, changes of temperature indoors, even by a few degrees, can intensify an attack.

Scientists are not certain why changes in temperature and humidity can have such a marked effect on asthma, though they warn us not to live near rivers or over underground streams in cities. These changes are closely bound up with the behaviour of the living allergens. Pollens are released in sunny weather, moulds in damp weather; and the seasons play their part. When the hay and corn are harvested, countless millions of mould spores are released into the air and drift over country and town alike. So the explanation as to why changes in the weather can affect asthma are many and various. The following ideas will at least illustrate some of the links between the two.

○ As was explained above in Chapter One, all our airways, upper and lower, are protected by a mucus blanket which is propelled upwards and outwards by tiny cilial hairs. In a dry atmosphere the blanket may disappear, exposing the sensitive tissues beneath. This is why central heating can contribute to wheeziness.

○ Cold air drives people indoors, where they are exposed to house dust mites and swap infections.

○ Moulds are active in warm damp weather. This is when they release their spores. Pollen grains open in damp weather and release their triggers.

○ Damp weather is associated with low clouds and these prevent polluted and pollen-laden air from rising. If at the same time the prevailing wind is blowing the smoke from a power station towards us, this can cause our airways to react.

○ We have seen that chest infections can trigger or worsen attacks of asthma. No less than 95 per cent of these are caused by virus colds, and these in turn are triggered by cold damp weather. The viruses live all the time in our upper breathing passages; it is the weather which causes them to multiply.

Why thunderstorms cause asthma

On 7 July 1983 a tremendous thunderstorm banged its way over Birmingham, England. Many with asthma were rushed into the hospitals, mostly between 9 p.m. and 6 a.m. There are many possible explanations for this. It might have been the drop in air pressure, or a 'temperature inversion' (warm air on top of cooler air) with zero wind speed and the airborne allergens unable to rise very far; there was a huge release of mould spores in the thundery rain flurries. Or it could have been a build-up in the atmosphere of oxides of nitrogen and of positive ions (discussed below). A recent explanation has emanated from Australia where it has been demonstrated that in damp and thundery weather pollen grains release particles which (unlike the grains themselves) are small enough to penetrate the smallest airways and trigger a response.

Ionizers and strange winds

In southern Europe in the summer, hot dry winds come from Africa which make people edgy and bad-tempered. In Bavaria there is a notorious wind which puts up the homicide rate. Scientists state that these winds are heavily charged with positive 'ions', tiny particles which can carry a positive or negative electrical charge. They also believe that positive ions can increase the amount of a hormone in the blood called serotonin, and that this is responsible for the ill effects, including a narrowing of the airways. These arguments are used commercially to support the sale of negative ionizers. Unfortunately, up to now, no one has been able to demonstrate that they do anything to prevent the attacks, possibly because they are too local in their output, but more probably because there are so many other trigger factors in asthma in addition to negative ions. It is best to try one out before buying it.

Fog and filthy air

Air pollution has been a trigger for asthma for many years. This was recognized by Sir John Floyer in 1698 in his treatise on asthma:

> Any kind of smoak offends the spirits of the Aſthmatic, and for that reaſon many of them cannot bear the Air of London, whoſe Smoak, like Fire it ſelf, irritates their Spirits into an Expanſion.

I well remember the 'pea-soupers', the smogs which affected our big cities before the Clean Air Act was passed in 1956 and created the smoke-free zones. The smog was a combination of dense fog and smoke, trapped close to the ground because of a sudden fall in temperature. The smoke came mainly from domestic coal fires and was responsible, during the great London smog of December 1952, for some 4,000 deaths from bronchitis and asthma (mainly the former).

Our present-day 'clean air' may be deceptive. Our power stations still fill the air with fumes (and can cover our shelves with a dark dust); lorries and motor cars pour forth noxious gases in ever increasing volumes; in the countryside farmers spray crops with toxic chemicals.

People with asthma do not welcome invitations to bonfire parties and barbecues and stay indoors when autumn leaves are being burned.

Below are listed just a few of the pollutants released into our atmosphere which can lead to symptoms of asthma.

Power stations

In the United Kingdom, oil- and coal-fired power stations are now responsible for three-quarters of the emissions of ***sulphur dioxide***. This is a gas which combines with water vapour in the air to form sulphuric acid, a powerful irritant. Some cities (for example Dublin and Athens) have high levels of ***particulates***, complex compounds, some of which are small enough to penetrate the small airways and are formed in the air from particles of sulphur dioxide and nitrogen oxide. If you have to live in a city, it is advisable to do so between the prevailing source of wind and the smoke-stacks. Gas-fired power stations are said to be less polluting than other kinds.

Motor vehicles

In the United Kingdom motor vehicles are the major source of ***nitrogen oxide*** in the atmosphere (followed by power stations). The vehicle emissions occur at near ground level and are highest in large conurbations near the kerbside during the rush-hour periods, a time to avoid when planning a visit to the high street shops.

Ozone

We all know about the protecting shield of ***ozone*** in the stratosphere. It diffuses down naturally to produce a background level on earth in the range 40–60 micrograms per cubic metre. At higher concentrations it can irritate the airways. It can increase to 300–700 mcgs/m^3 as a result of 'photochemical smog', when nitrogen oxides and hydrocarbons from vehicles and power stations combine with sunlight to form ozone and other irritant gases such as hydrogen peroxide. It was originally thought that this was a problem only in Los Angeles, but in polluted air in Europe maximum 1-hour ozone levels may exceed 350 mcgs/m^3 in the cities. This is especially likely in an anti-cyclone when there is plenty of sunshine and a temperature inversion which stops upper and lower air from mixing.

The need for research

There has been surprisingly little research into the links between atmospheric pollution and asthma. This is partly because there are only a few monitoring stations, partly because it is hard to isolate the triggers one from another and partly because each locality is unique in its ability to generate harmful emissions. Links between irritant gases and asthma have however been clearly demonstrated in laboratories and on the ground, and it seems possible that the rising incidence of asthma may be due, at least in part, to increasing levels of air pollution. The gases not only trigger short-term asthma, they can increase sensitivity to allergens in general.

No smoking please!

Not only do we poison the air outside our homes and offices but quite often pollute the interior as well. Many people with asthma find that cigar and cigarette smoke is the worst form of air pollution. Their airways are exquisitely sensitive to the many different chemicals generated by smouldering tobacco.

It is now clear that an increase in smoking among pregnant women is contributing to an increase in asthma in children; it appears to upset the development of a child's immune system. Passive smoking may contribute to this after a child has been born and can interfere with normal lung development. Once sensitized, the smoke becomes a trigger for asthma attacks.

In addition, smoking may make people exposed to allergens at work more likely to respond to them. One famous example is sensitivity to the unloading of soya flour in the docks at Barcelona: it is the smokers who are allergic to the flour who are most affected by it (see page 72).

Many people with asthma do smoke, either to calm their nerves or because the smoke stimulates the mucus glands and helps them cough up the phlegm. They may not be aware that the smoke also paralyses the cilia which are designed to clear the mucus blanket and helps to disrupt the protective lining of the airways and exposes them to an attack by viruses.

As a result, the lungs become less and less able to defend themselves against invading bacteria, even with antibiotics, so that in time the air sacs (alveoli) are damaged. This is the condition known as ***chronic bronchitis***. It is not reversible and fills hospital beds with people whose lives have become miserable indeed.

Giving up smoking

How this is done is beyond the scope of this book, but useful advice can be obtained from the Health Education Authority and from A.S.H., whose addresses are given at the end of the book. There are four stages in the process of giving up smoking:

1 think of all the reasons for stopping
2 decide how smoking is linked to certain habits
3 choose a BIG DAY and cut out smoking altogether
4 do not slip back, and reward success by giving yourself and your family a treat with the money you have saved.

If you are an employer who wants to impose a ban on smoking there are three rules you must bear in mind: consult the workforce; announce and publicize the policy in advance; and make emergency arrangements for smokers who cannot give up immediately.

There is an alternative to smoking. About a million people in Britain now take snuff. This habit does no damage to the lungs or to the nasal passages and apparently provides uplift. Chewing gum containing nicotine is another alternative to smoking.

Changing attitudes to smoking

The campaign by the anti-smoking lobby is gathering strength. Smoking is increasingly being banned from public transport and from centres which the public is required to attend. This has gained encouragement from a court action in Australia. A woman claimed that thirteen years' exposure to tobacco smoke at a Sydney health centre had undermined her health. She was awarded £35,000 in damages. A less drastic step would be to write to your Member of Parliament or to send a letter to the local newspaper, complaining about smoking in premises used by the public.

Barcelona revisited

Barcelona is a busy port, surrounded by hills. From 1981 onwards epidemics of severe asthma broke out among the local population from time to time. These were limited to a small area and occurred over a few hours. It took six years to find out what was responsible, and the answer throws a beam of light on the way asthma can develop.

It was already known that onshore breezes meeting a circle of hills can lead to cool air lying trapped under warm air, causing any pollutants to remain near the ground. It was also clear that one very specific trigger was responsible. Smoke from outbreaks of fire was ruled out. The unloading of castor beans, a powerful trigger for asthma, in the port was eliminated.

Blood samples of those affected were kept and frozen over the years, and in 1987 these were tested to see which of a whole range of triggers provoked an antibody reaction. Soya bean flour was included, and this proved to be the culprit. When loaded into silos the dust had escaped and, in the special weather conditions described (as checked by weather records matched against the movements of cargo vessels), descended and caused asthma in people who had never had attacks before. Filters were added to the silos and the attacks ceased.

The attacks started a year after the first shipment of soya flour arrived: the time usually taken for people to develop sensitivities. They were confined to adults, and smokers were especially likely to be affected. The story also reminds us that about 40 per cent of people carry a gene which, given a suitable combination of challenges, can allow asthma to appear for the first time. The story can act as a summary of the previous sections in this chapter.

Where should we live?

Now and again I meet people who tell me that their asthma has been transformed when they moved house, either from the town to the country or the other way round. In my own case it became markedly worse when I moved a few miles from a third-floor flat in Kensington, London, to a house near the busy New King's Road. I think I would prefer an island in the Mediteranean; but Napoleon suffered from asthma when exiled to Elba.

The scientists assure us that the prevalence of asthma is broadly similar in areas of the United Kingdom as far apart as London, the Midlands, Wales, the North-east and Scotland. Of greater importance are local factors. I have not found local authorities able to give much guidance but they will explain if there are any underground rivers, to cause extra damp. A large-scale map will show the way the prevailing wind is likely to spread pollution from power stations, major factories and busy roads. River valleys are often said to be bad for asthma; but most towns are built in them! The type of house is important. Some houses, when they cool, develop more condensation than others – high levels of humidity favour moulds and mites.

Some drugs can cause asthma

It is not generally realized that some drugs can cause severe asthma. One group of these is connected with aspirin, and sensitivity to aspirin is especially associated with those asthmatics who also develop nasal polyps. Many drugs which can be bought over the counter for colds, headaches and rheumatism contain aspirin; an asthmatic who is sensitive to aspirin should consult the retail pharmacist before making a purchase, and check the chemical names on any bottle of pain reliever (acetylsalicylic acid and salicylate = aspirin). Some NSAIDs (non-steroidal anti-inflammatory drugs), for example 'Ibuprofen' and

'Indomethacin' (which is used for severe back pain), can also cause severe asthma in aspirin-sensitive people.

Among the many drugs used to treat high blood pressure, there is a group called the 'beta-blocker' drugs. These can initiate asthma in people who react to them, and the resultant illness can be so severe as to cause death. Eye-drops containing a beta-blocker, sometimes used in cases of glaucoma, for example Timoptol, should also be avoided since there have been cases of death being caused by asthma following the placing of a single drop in each eye. Pylocarpine does not carry this risk.

Chemicals and additives

Some people with asthma find that their asthma gets worse when the walls of their home have just been painted and are giving off solvent fumes; water-based paint would avoid this. Other chemicals used in the home which can make some people with asthma wheeze include air-fresheners, hair sprays, talcum powder, and washing powder which contains enzymes. The perfumes now used in many household cleaning products can cause distress. Solvents are used not only to thin paints, in the form of white spirit, but are also used in dry-cleaning and carpet-cleaning fluids and in many glues. Dieldrin mothproofer is released by solvents, and wood preservatives based on Lindane or PLP produce a vapour which can cause wheeziness. (It is alarming to read that some solvents can react to the flames from a gas fire to produce phosgene gas!) Escaping gas can cause asthma: make sure the pilot light on the cooker is kept lit. Faulty boiler flues need attention.

It can happen that a person with only mild or latent asthma can be overwhelmed by exposure to a chemical additive and from then on become much more responsive to the other triggers. Some chemicals are hidden but can still cause trouble, for example formaldehyde in chipboard used by the office furniture industry. Some local authorities provide an environmental health service, which includes a Home Check Scheme designed to point out possible health hazards.

There is increasing concern that latex, used for domestic and surgical gloves and condoms, may cause an allergic reaction, especially if the newer formulations are provided.

A particularly distressing form of asthma is that which arises directly from a person's occupation, for example in the bakery trade or as a hairdresser. This is discussed on page 203. Mothers of children with asthma often worry about the many chemical additives which now find their way into our manufactured foods, a topic which is treated in Chapter Eleven.

Infections

It is a common experience among people with asthma that coughs and colds make their asthma worse – indeed, may provoke an attack in the first place. Some people have asthma only when they have a cold, or at least they believe this to be the case.

The cold is typically caused by a rhinovirus ('rhino' being a medical term for the nose). These viruses can easily descend to the breathing tubes and act as irritants, or they may contribute to the breakdown of the linings of the breathing tubes if there is a severe infection. The presence of viruses can make the airways more 'twitchy', more responsive to other irritants.

Bacteria may arrive as well; and these can stimulate the production of antibodies, as well as producing histamine themselves. There may be present, especially in older people, a bronchitis which causes the production of phlegm and it is often difficult for either doctor or patient to decide whether it is the asthma or the bronchitis which is the major cause of phlegm.

Infection is particularly likely to precipitate asthma in infants and young children with the syncytial virus predominating, and in older adults. Feverish, influenza-like illnesses which do not have the symptoms of a head cold are generally less provoking.

Other infections such as measles, chicken-pox and diarrhoea do not trigger attacks of asthma.

It is important for the distinction between 'asthma' and various forms of bronchitis to be made clear to the patient. 'Wheezy bronchitis' is just another name for asthma, but one which may conceal the true nature of the illness.

Doctors sometimes prescribe an antibiotic when there is an infection. This is not aimed at the virus, against which it is powerless, nor will it directly lessen the asthmatic response. It is aimed at the secondary infection which can, as we have seen, trigger this response. This argument is taken further in Chapter Four, 'Other medicines', on page 106.

Some parents take the idealistic view that they should try to shield their children completely from exposure to infections. This is clearly impossible, especially when the child starts going to school. On the contrary, school games and exercises are essential in the achievement of physical fitness, and this, together with warm clothes and a balanced diet, will help build resistance to the viruses. If the head colds are very numerous, then allergic rhinitis may be suspected and should be treated as such.

As someone with severe asthma, I take the precaution of avoiding going into crowded places such as theatres and cinemas in the months when they are likely to attract people full of coughs and sneezes, since I find I pick up infection very easily, and changes in temperature, from cold street to warm theatre, can encourage the cold viruses. In adults, asthma can be provoked by Influenza 'A' virus, so if you have severe chronic asthma it is a good plan to ask your doctor to inoculate you against influenza in October or November when the vaccine becomes available.

Asthma at night

Many people with asthma find that it is worse at night or when waking, usually after 3 a.m. This is often referred to as 'the early morning dip', that is to say, a dip in the reading of peak flow, as described on page 143. Night asthma is a major cause of hospital referrals in asthma, and loss of sleep affects performance during the following day. Why does it take place? Various theories have been put forward:

o In the seventeenth century Sir Thomas Willis ascribed it to 'an overheating of the blood by the bed clothes'. Nowadays physicians know that the blood temperature remains constant, but they are aware that the house dust mite likes to live in bed linen (especially in wool and feathers), and to feed on the tiny skin scales which humans shed at night. But many asthmatics who are not allergic to house dust mite nevertheless have night asthma, so there must be some additional explanation.

o Another factor could be the 'late allergic reaction' described in the last chapter. But not all asthmatics are allergic and second-phase attacks are not nearly as common as night asthma.

o It is tempting to suppose that night asthma is simply due to the fact that the aerosol bronchodilator taken at 11 p.m. has no effect after 3 a.m. But some patients wheeze in the early hours even when a bronchodilator is used which releases the medicine slowly throughout the night.

o At night, the clearance of mucus through the beating of the cilia in the airways decreases markedly during sleep, so there is likely to be a build-up of allergens and irritants in the mucus. This may contribute, but it is not believed to be the major factor. Scientists also view the cooling of the airways at night to be too slight to be significant, especially when the room temperature is well maintained.

o Until recently it was thought that the changes in the supply of hormones which take place at night (they drop just as the peak flow drops), especially corticosteroids, could explain night asthma. However, these hormones are made by the adrenal glands, and in asthmatics the drop in peak flow still takes place even when the glands have been removed (for other reasons).

There remains one possible explanation: that sleep itself is the cause of night asthma. In 1698 Sir John Floyer seems to have had the same opinion: 'I have observed,' he wrote, 'that Fits of Asthma seem always to happen after Sleep in the Night, when the nerves are filled with windy Spirits.' It has been shown in shift workers that the time their airways narrow is when they are asleep, and this has been reproduced in studies in which asthmatics are kept awake one night and allowed to sleep the next.

It is not a 'windy spirit' which is responsible but the circadian (around-the-clock) rhythm. In every human being, sleep brings with it a slight reduction in the heart rate, in blood pressure and in the diameter of the airways. In people with asthma these narrow to a much greater extent, and they start from a lower level anyway.

In Chapter Five we will see that if ***peak flow*** falls, as between day time and night time, by more than 15 per cent then this is a sign that the asthma is not well controlled and ***preventive*** medicine is indicated. If this fails to eliminate the night-time asthma,then a slow-release **reliever** may be suggested by the medical team (see pages 93 and 96).

The triggers: a summary

Thirty years ago, before many of the present medicines were developed, great attention was paid to ways of avoiding or reducing triggers, esecially those in the home. This diminished with the wave of new medicines, introduced in the 1970s and '80s.

Today there is renewed interest in the triggers, partly because the medicines have not halted the rising incidence of asthma, partly because of widespread concern about the environment and partly because there is a growing understanding of the way the triggers act.

Before leaving this subject, we should distinguish between triggers which make asthma worse and those which cause attacks but do not usually change the underlying sensitivity of the airways.

Triggers that make underlying asthma worse

allergens	**pollen, house dust, animals, moulds**
infections	**syncytial virus, rhinovirus (colds)**
triggers at work	**isocyanates, platinum salts etc.**

Triggers that cause attacks but do not make asthma worse

breathing	**exercise, over-breathing, cold air**
airborne chemicals	**sulphur dioxide, ozone, passive tobacco smoke, solvents used in the home**
emotional	**upsets, excitement, auto-suggestion**

CHAPTER FOUR

A Wide Choice of Medicines

Arranging them in 'families'

The aim of treatment should be that every person with asthma can remain free from symptoms at all times and able to lead a normal life. A secondary aim is that this should be achieved without fear of side-effects.

Unfortunately, this aim cannot be achieved for everyone, with the present range of medicines. On the other hand, many sufferers would enjoy a much greater degree of relief if they were able to understand what each remedy aims to achieve and to use what has been prescribed to the best advantage.

For the purpose of this chapter, the medicines currently fall into four groups. The '**relievers**' aim to open up the airways when they have tightened during an attack. They are taken as needed. The '**protectors**' aim to keep the airways open for a longer period than the relievers and are taken on a regular basis. The '**preventers**' will not reverse an attack by relaxing the airway muscles. They act to damp down inflammation, the underlying cause of asthma, over a much longer period of time and are taken each day. In a very severe attack, which does not respond to the relievers, then there is a choice of '**acute savers**'; some of these are reserved for the doctor's use.

How does the doctor choose the treatment?

Having diagnosed that you are suffering from asthma, the doctor proceeds as follows. He at first prescribes the lowest dose and

Group A: **Relievers** (*swords*) †

aim: to relax the airway muscles

bronchodilators derivatives of:

A1 *adrenaline* (e.g. Aerolin, Berotec, Bricanyl, Ventolin)

A2 *caffeine* (many brands of theophylline)

A3 *atropine* (e.g. Atrovent, Duovent, Oxivent)

Group B: **Protectors** (*shields*) ⊗

aim: to keep the airway muscles relaxed

B1 *salmeterol* (Serevent)

B2 *bambuterol* (Bambec)

Group C: **Preventers** (*shields*) ⊗

aim: to prevent a build up of inflammation

anti-inflammatory

C1 inhaled steroids (e.g. Aerobec, Becotide, Becloforte, Filair, Flixotide, Pulmicort)

C2 non-steroidal, anti-allergic (e.g. Aerocrom, Intal, Tilade)

anti-allergic

C3 anti-histamine (e.g. Zaditen)

Group D: **Acute savers** (*swords*) †

aim: to relieve a severe attack with high doses of:

D1 tablet steroids (e.g. Prednisolone)

D2 bronchodilators (especially A1)

simplest treatment that seems to fit the kind of asthma that has been presented.

This treatment may be successful. On the other hand, you may return to the surgery a few weeks later and complain that the symptoms still occur. This may be due to one or more of the following reasons:

- o the medicine was not taken correctly (see especially the section on inhalers on page 111)
- o it was used properly, but you worried about possible side-effects and gave up
- o the form in which the medicine was taken was not suitable. Medicines can be taken in many ways: they can be swallowed as syrups or tablets; inhaled as a powder or as droplets from a breath-operated inhaler
- o the medicine failed to relieve symptoms at night
- o the medicine relieved the asthma for a few hours but the dose then had to be repeated because symptoms returned

No two patients are alike

Doctors soon recognize that no two patients are alike in the way they respond to the medicines. This is because people vary in their ability to absorb the drugs and, hence, the degree to which the drugs will cause side-effects.

People also vary in their present understanding of the illness and the extent to which they feel able to comply with the instructions they have been given. It follows that doctors have to proceed very largely by *trial and error.*

Modern medicines are 'safe'

Nearly all effective medicines have 'side-effects': they cause reactions in the body which by themselves do not bring the required benefit. We must not confuse side-effects which are dangerous with those that are merely unpleasant. Some of the medicines used to treat asthma can cause reactions which are upsetting, for example a tremor in the hands. These reactions are not necessarily dangerous.

As far as safety is concerned, we should distinguish between the remedies available up to the 1970s and those which have been introduced since. Before the 1970s, we had theophylline, which starts to be harmful at about twice the treatment dose. There was isoprenaline, which upsets heart rhythms, and we had tablet steroids, which, if taken in high doses over long periods, can have debilitating effects. Since that time, a safer slow-release theophylline has appeared; isoprenaline has been superseded by selective airway dilators which do not act on the heart muscles to the same extent; inhaled steroids have replaced tablet steroids, except in crisis management.

'Can I take more than one medicine at a time, or will this increase the toxic effects?' The opposite may be the case, because it may be possible to reduce the dose of one type of drug if another is used as well, assuming that they operate through different routes to bring relief. On the other hand it is best to avoid taking more than, say, three remedies.

They are not addictive

None of the treatments is a drug of addiction in the sense in which tranquillizers have this potential. However, recent research into the relievers suggests that you should use them only as needed and not on a regular, 'four times a day' basis that used to be prescribed. Preventive treatment may often be needed as well, as described later in this chapter.

Some parents believe that their teenage children have become addicted to the propellant used in aerosol inhalers. This is unlikely, but the remedy would be to switch to a powder-based inhaler.

What is meant by the 'placebo' effect?

Some asthmatics react favourably to treatments which have no proven therapeutic value. Such treatments are said to have a 'placebo' effect as, for example, when inert substances are given in clinical trials as a means of comparing the response when active drugs are used. This suggests that there are asthmatics, clearly a minority, in whom the power of suggestion is strong, and this is one of the reasons why doctors may be reluctant to change a course of treatment which has become out-dated, if the patient feels benefit from it. The converse is also true: that if for any reason a patient resents the treatment that has been prescribed, it is unlikely to be fully effective, even though backed by the evidence of numerous clinical trials.

How are the drugs given?

This will be discussed in more detail in 'A closer look at the inhalers' on page 111. For our present purposes, the methods available can be divided quite simply into two general types:

	Taken at home	*Given only by the doctor*
The drug circulates in the bloodstream	**tablets** **capsules** **syrups**	**injections**
The drug is inhaled into the air passages	**aerosols** **powders**	

Each method has its advantages and disadvantages. If the drug has to circulate round the bloodstream before it reaches the air passages, it will enter all parts of the body and produce responses where they are not needed. On the other hand, if the air passages are blocked, this may be the most effective route. Tablets can be modified to provide slow release of the drug over an extended period, and this can help relieve night-time attacks.

It is generally more effective to deliver the drug directly to the air passages by inhaling it, and any side-effects are likely to be greatly reduced thereby. Drugs act much more quickly when inhaled than when swallowed as tablets. To increase the effectiveness, a device such as a spacer can be fitted to the inhaler. To deal with a severe attack, the doctor can inject a large dose via the bloodstream or use a nebulizer, which enables a continuous stream of fine particles of the drug to be inhaled.

When choosing between these methods, the doctor has to take into account the age of the patient, the type of asthma, the probable triggers and the seriousness of the attacks. The patient's own preferences also have to be considered. At first the wide choice of routes and devices can seem bewildering, but there is one great advantage: if one method fails to give relief then another can be tried, so the patient should never give up but insist that an effective method be found.

Relievers and protectors

Group A: **Relievers (*bronchodilators*)** †

The aim: to relax the smooth muscle which surrounds the air passages (*bronchi*) so as to relieve the **bronchospasm**. Recent research has confirmed that most bronchodilators have little or no effect on the inflammation in the airways which underlies asthma (see 'Preventers', below).

There is a wide choice of bronchodilators, each available in many forms. They divide into three groups:

A1: derived from adrenaline
salbutamol (Ventolin, Volmax, Aerolin, Salbulin)
terbutaline (Bricanyl)
fenoterol (Berotec)

procaterol (Pro-Air, not available in the U.K.)
pirbuterol (Maxair, not available in the U.K.)

A2: derived from caffeine
aminophylline (Phyllocontin)
theophylline (Nuelin, Slo-Phyllin, Theo-Dur)

A3: derived from atropine
ipratropium (Atrovent, Duovent)
oxitropium (Oxivent)

A1 Bronchodilators derived from adrenaline †

Before the Second World War, adrenaline (given by injection) and ephedrine (taken as a tablet) were the only drugs available for relieving an asthma attack. They did so, very effectively, by reversing spasm of the muscles surrounding the airways. Unfortunately they had undesirable effects as well: a racing pulse, anxiety and excitement.

Scientists in the pharmaceutical companies spent a lot of time looking for derivatives of adrenaline which would relieve spasm of the airway muscles without stimulating the heart muscles. Their first achievement was to bring out an aerosol inhaler with metered doses which was more efficient than the old bulb inhaler. Unfortunately the drug available at the time, isoprenaline, stimulated the heart as well.

The big breakthrough came when new airway-dilating drugs were developed which latched on to the Beta-2 receptors in the airway muscles but which had only a small effect on the receptors in the heart muscles. They are often referred to as 'Beta-2 agonists' or 'sympathomimetic' agents because they stimulate that part of the sympathetic nervous system which dilates the airways. The brands which are used most commonly in the United Kingdom, Australia and New Zealand are (in alphabetical order) Aerolin, Berotec, Bricanyl and Ventolin.

This group of drugs only relieves muscle spasm in the airways and does not reduce inflammation or reduce the 'twitchiness' (the way the airways respond over time to irritants). This is why they are called 'relievers'. However, when taken 10–20 minutes before exercise or exposure to cold air, they act to prevent airway muscle spasm on a short-term basis.

Their second disadvantage is that, when used on their own, at high doses and on a regular daily basis, the Beta-2 agonist relievers can, in time, become less and less effective. This is likely to happen only if more than ten puffs a day are taken. It seems that the Beta-2 receptors in the airway become fewer so that the drug can no longer act on them efficiently. This was first suggested in New Zealand for fenoterol and was confirmed later by trials in Saskatchewan in Canada. Very recent research in Glasgow suggests that, at repeated high doses of Beta-2 agonists, a hormone called angiotensin is released during attacks of asthma and this can make the attacks worse.

So the rule now is to reserve high doses of reliever for the occasional severe attack and take a reliever **only as needed. If required more frequently than once a day or three times a week, a preventer should be used in addition.**

In a very severe attack it may be desirable to take 30 to 40 puffs of the reliever (Ventolin, Berotec, Bricanyl, or Aerolin), preferably through a large spacer (see page 115). This is a 'one-off' procedure; if you have a heart condition, check first with your doctor that this will be appropriate.

How are they taken?

There are various ways in which these adrenaline derivatives can be taken at home. They can be swallowed as syrups, or as tablets which can incorporate a slow-release facility. They can be inhaled as dry powders or with aerosol sprays; the sprays can be provided with tube spacers or large volume spacers. They can be inhaled from nebulizers which are driven by compressed air. These forms are available for other medicines used in asthma; their function will be described in Chapter Five. The doctor has an additional route for administration: he can inject directly into the bloodstream, under the skin or into a muscle. But it is now more common for a doctor to use a nebulizer to give a high dose in an acute attack.

Inhalers: advantages and disadvantages

Bronchodilators taken from an inhaler have advantages over syrups and tablets. They act directly on the airways; as a result, they act quickly, within five minutes, and only a tiny dose is needed. This is measured in micrograms (μg.) or one-thousandth part of a milligram. The dose can be repeated when needed to relieve wheeziness. (See the table on the next page for a comparison of doses of salbutamol delivered in various ways.)

Side-effects are minimal: some people experience what they call 'the shakes': a trembling of the hands which wears off after a few minutes. At higher doses the pulse-rate may quicken and the heart may start to pound. These symptoms are unpleasant but not dangerous. Older people with a heart condition should consult their doctor if they occur.

There are disadvantages. Conventional metered-dose inhalers propelled by an aerosol need a co-ordination between squeeze and breathing which young children and arthritic people can find difficult. This can be partly overcome by adding a special lever to the inhaler. Better still, we can use a device which releases the spray when we breathe inwards (the Autohaler). An alternative is to use one of the dry powder inhalers, for example the Turbohaler, because these too are activated by an in-drawing of breath. All these devices are described in Chapter Five.

The second disadvantage is that the dose, however taken, lasts for only 4–5 hours. This can be remedied with tablet forms such as Volmax and Bricanyl SA which release the medicine slowly, or by using slow-release theophyllines, or one of the new protectors (Serevent or Bambec) described below.

How doses compare when taken in different ways

(*Ventolin is given as an example*)

form	*size of dose per tablet or puff or nebule*	*doses which are generally recommended*			
		age	*dose*	*times a day*	*maximum in 24 hours*
('oral route')					
tablet	2 mg. or 4 mg.	infant	nil		
		2–6 years	1–2 mg.	3 or 4	
syrup		6–12 years	2 mg.		
		adult	2–4 mg.	up to 4	16 mg.
slow-release tablet*	8 mg.	child	nil		
		adult	1	up to 2	16 mg.
metered-dose aerosol inhaler (as used for regular treatment)	100 μg.	child	½ adult		
		adult	up to 2 puffs	as needed	
inhaled powder**	200 μg.	child	½ adult		
		adult	up to 2 puffs	as needed	
nebulizer	2.5–5 mg.	adult	1–2 nebules	4-hourly	20 mg.
injection (subcutaneous or intramuscular)	500 mg.	(dose relates to body weight)		4-hourly	

* Volmax ** Rotacaps

The size of the doses discharged may be compared in the following chart:

10 mg. by nebulizer = 100 times
4 mg. by oral tablet = 40 times
400 μg. by Rotacap = 4 times
} the amount discharged by inhaler (100 μg.)

1,000 micrograms (μg.) = 1 milligram (mg.)

The third disadvantage is that many forget that metered-dose aerosol inhalers take 30 seconds to recharge, and this requires some patience! Two puffs in quick succession are not appropriate. I use two inhalers.

A fourth problem is that the freon propellant is a chlorofluorocarbon (C.F.C.) and the Montreal Agreement sets a timetable for phasing out C.F.C.s by 1997. It is possible that C.F.C.s used in medicine will be exempt; or that C.F.C.s will be recycled from old refrigerators; new ways of nebulizing (or the Brovon spray system) may be developed; new propellants are being developed. Dry powder inhalers provide an alternative.

Spacers and nebulizers

These will be compared in the next chapter. Until quite recently nebulizers were widely recommended for patients with moderately severe asthma to relieve attacks, using a reliever (bronchodilator) such as salbutamol or terbutaline. Nowadays doctors are more likely to prescribe a large-volume spacer instead. They are cheaper, easier and faster, and they are portable. They can be just as effective in delivering the bronchodilator in the form of a fine vapour, even when the breathing is restricted (see page 115).

As far as relievers are concerned, nebulizers tend to be restricted to children and adults who have severe asthma.

Adrenaline derivatives: a summary

This group forms the first line of defence. People with mild asthma may need no other treatment. This is usually via a blue pocket inhaler which is carried around at all times, with reserve inhalers placed in strategic places, such as in the glove compartment of the car, under the pillow and in a drawer at the office.

These bronchodilators act fast to relieve airway constriction, however caused. Though there is a warning on the pack which says 'it is dangerous to exceed the stated dose', the adrenaline derivatives are not dangerous. However, if they are required more than once a day or more than three days a week, then preventive medicine is needed as well. They are not used on a regular basis, but only as required to bring relief.

There are **three important rules** to observe:

o Learn how to use the inhaler correctly so that you get enough medicine into the lungs; for example, always shake the device before each puff (see page 113)

Some common brand names in various countries (adrenaline derivatives)

	U.K.	U.S.A.	Canada	Australia	New Zealand
salbutamol					
Ventolin	√	√	√	√	√
Volmax	√	×	√	×	√
Aerolin Autohaler	√	×	×	*Respolin*	*Respolin*
Salbulin	√	×	×	×	×
terbutaline					
Bricanyl	√	×	√	√	√
fenoterol					
Berotec	√	×	×	√	√
Berodual	×	√	√	×	×
procaterol					
Pro Air	×	√			
pirbuterol					
Maxair	×	√			

√ listed in 1993 blanks indicate lack of data
× not listed in 1993

N.B. The countries chosen are those in which this book is distributed.

○ Use the inhaler as soon as you feel an attack coming on

○ Take the dose as prescribed. If this does not bring relief, seek fresh medical advice (see especially the section in Chapter Six on 'What to do if things go wrong', page 136). In a *crisis*, up to 40 puffs can be taken: but check with your doctor that this is suitable for you

A2 Relievers derived from caffeine† (xanthines)

Theophylline occurs naturally in tea and coffee and is closely related to coffee. It has been said that the stimulating action of coffee was first discovered by an Arabian monk who noticed that the goats which had eaten berries from coffee plants became frisky. Coffee and extracts from tea plants have been used to treat asthma for 700 years, but only in the twentieth century has the active substance, theophylline, been identified. Aminophylline, a soluble form of the same drug, is used by injection if there is a severe attack.

Like the adrenaline derivatives described above, theophylline is prescribed solely to *relieve* spasm of the airway muscles; it relaxes them and probably stimulates the body's own production of adrenaline. It is not designed to *prevent* inflammation.

The toxic hazards

Theophylline has two main disadvantages. It cannot be taken from an inhaler because this causes coughing, which makes the asthma worse. The second problem is that it is not selective and affects not only the breathing tubes but also the heart, brain, kidneys and stomach. These disturbances start to become troublesome at only twice the dose used for relieving asthma. Some patients cannot tolerate it at all, even in very small doses. The theophylline drugs are not recommended for young children.

Others find they can obtain relief at a dosage which does not produce the nausea, the stomach pains, the headache, the sleepless nights and the emotional disturbance (elation followed by depression).

The toxicity varies according to when a meal was last taken, and it is affected by cigarette smoking. It also varies according to the level in the blood, and this should be checked from time to time; too high a level could be dangerous and the dosage may need to be reduced. Some drugs, used to treat other illnesses, can increase the toxicity of theophylline; these include an antibiotic (erythromycin) and a drug to relieve stomach ulcers (cimetidine). Clearance of the drug from the system can also be delayed by infections and the use of oral contraceptives.

If medical help is sought during a crisis attack, always tell the doctor if theophylline or aminophylline have been taken, to avoid a dangerous double-dosing. Any asthmatic on one of these drugs should take no higher dose than has been prescribed and should avoid all over-the-counter preparations such as Do Do or Franolyn Expect, which also contain theophylline. The retail pharmacist will advise what these are.

On the continent, but no longer in the U.K., aminophylline is available as a suppository. This reduces the risk of an upset stomach and can bring fast relief from a severe attack, but it can cause bowel irritation and the size of the dose which is absorbed is unpredictable.

Slow-release forms have advantages

In spite of all these disadvantages, remedies based on theophylline are still widely prescribed in some countries, especially in North America. They had a new lease of life when slow-release forms began to appear. One way in which this is achieved is to store the particles of drug in a miniature wax honeycomb which is encased in a plastic coating. This is gradually removed by the bile acid so that the drug is slowly absorbed from the intestine. Brand names of the slow-release theophyllines include

Nuelin SA, Slo-Phyllin, Sabidal SR, Theo-Dur and Uniphyllin. Some of these slow-release forms can provide a twenty-four-hour cover with only two doses and so help prevent night asthma (see the table, below). Some brands, such as Phyllocontin, have tablets designed for children.

Theophylline: a table of brands

	when taken	**Brand names** U.K.	**Brand names** U.S.A and Canada
Short-acting (2–4 hours)	every 4–6 hours	Aminophylline Bronchodil	Elixophyllin Quibron Somophyllin
Medium-acting (4–8 hours)	every 8 hours	Nuelin Slo-Phyllin Sabidal SR	Theolair SR Theophyl SR
Longer-acting (over 8 hours)	twice a day	Theo-Dur Uniphyllin Phyllocontin Continus	Constant-T Slo-Bid Theo-Dur Uniphyl

SR = slow-release

A3 Atropine derivatives † (anti-cholinergics)

In childhood my first introduction to any kind of medicine for asthma was the once-famous 'Potter's Asthma Cure', described on page 12. It consisted of inhaling the smoke from the burning leaves of stramonium. A few years later I was taken to an ancient herbalist who lived in a dark basement; she examined the specimen I had brought and added powders which gave rise to brightly coloured exhalations. She muttered mysteriously and, when a fee had been produced and accepted, dived into a cupboard and produced a liquid not unlike, in appearance, that which I had provided and in a similar corked bottle. It turned out to be belladonna.

Belladonna is extracted from the plant *Atropa Belladonna*, more commonly known as deadly nightshade. Fashionable ladies used to take a tincture as eye-drops to dilate their pupils, hence the name of the plant.

A modern derivative of atropine, **ipratropium**, is prescribed today. It is used only from an inhaler or nebulizer and it has a bitter taste. There are two brand names: Atrovent and Duovent. Duovent is a combination of ipratropium and fenoterol, the idea being that the dose of each can be reduced when they are added together. The rule about 'only used as needed' does not apply – this reliever is taken four times a day.

The aim is to relax the bronchial muscles when they are constricting the airways; Atrovent does this by blocking the vagus nerve. Side-effects are few; when Atrovent is nebulized with a large dose, the mouth may become dry. Patients with glaucoma should avoid allowing the spray to reach the eyes.

As a bronchodilator, Atrovent is generally no better than Ventolin and Bricanyl. Why is it used?

- in infants, when it is nebulized, it can be more effective than the other bronchodilators
- it is useful in chronic bronchitis which in older people may be mixed with asthma
- it is useful for people who find that other relievers (salbutamol and terbutaline) give them 'the shakes'
- it can be mixed with salbutamol and nebulized to relieve a severe attack

Oxitropium is a similar drug, but with a longer duration, and is used twice a day on a regular basis. The brand name is Oxivent.

Atrovent is available in the U.K., U.S.A., Canada and New Zealand, and (restricted to ampoules for nebulizers) in Australia.

Oxivent and Duovent are available in the U.K. and in New Zealand.

Group B: **Protectors** ⊗

'Protectors' have been introduced recently. They are *relievers* in that they relax the airway muscles. They do not bring immediate relief but instead act on the muscles with continuous and constant doses over extended periods of time. This why some writers like to refer to them as *protectors*.

Protectors are an add-on treatment: they are prescribed only when *preventers* (inhaled steroids or Intal) are used in addition. Short-term *relievers* (Ventolin or Bricanyl) continue to be taken as needed to reverse attacks as they take place. Another characteristic of protectors is that, to be effective, they have to be used on a regular basis. They take time to become established, so do not give up if there is no immediate improvement.

Protectors are especially indicated when symptoms such as night cough persist in spite of regular treatment with inhaled steroids or Intal. The *aim* is to raise early morning peak flow readings closer to the evening levels (see page 150) and help prevent sleep disturbance. A secondary effect may be that evening levels improve as well.

The side-effects of the protectors are those associated with Ventolin and Bricanyl: a mild tremor, headache and palpitations in some patients. These are not dangerous and lessen as the treatment continues. They do not cause problems unless the recommended dose is exceeded. Protectors should not be used in association with the theophyllines.

BI **Salmeterol** ⊗

Salmeterol is like Ventolin and Bricanyl in that it latches on to the Beta-2 receptors in the airway muscles. The difference is that it has a long molecular tail which provides a stable anchor.

Serevent lasts for 12 hours and, if taken twice daily, gives round-the-clock protection.

Salmeterol (brand name Serevent) is taken in a dose of 50 micrograms twice daily. This can be increased to 100 micrograms in adults. It is administered from a green aerosol inhaler (25 micrograms per actuation) or in powder form from a Diskhaler (50 micrograms). The aerosol tends to make you catch your breath momentarily.

Serevent can be used by adults, and by children over four years of age. As far as parents are concerned, the dosage is simple, and protection is provided from a single dose throughout the school day, offering a defence against exercise-induced asthma.

B2 Bambuterol ⊗

Bambuterol (brand name Bambec) is a 'pro-drug' of terbutaline. This means that it is broken down ('metabolized') slowly and transformed into terbutaline (Bricanyl). By this means it provides a continuous dose of *relieving* medicine over 24 hours. At the time of writing, it is only used in adults, but will no doubt be extended to children in due course.

Bambec was introduced in 1993 into the U.K. and is taken as a 10 mg. tablet from a blister pack once a day, preferably in the evening. If necessary the dose can be increased to 20 mg. a day. Like Bricanyl SA (slow-release) it has to be in the form of a tablet and would not work if provided from an inhaler. It is suitable for elderly patients at the full dose.

Preventers ⊗

Group C: **Anti-inflammatory agents**

C1 Inhaled steroids ⊗

In the last few years it has been realized that air passages may be inflamed even in mild asthma. To reduce and then prevent inflammation, a quite different kind of treatment is needed compared with the *relievers*.

The most commonly prescribed anti-inflammatory agents are the inhaled steroids. These are powerful drugs. It is no exaggeration to say that they have transformed the treatment of asthma when it is due to inflammation of the tissues surrounding the airways. They may be described as *preventers*.

They act at many cellular levels to damp down inflammation. For example, they help to block the release of mediators from the mast cells and they help prevent lymphocytes from becoming active (see page 31). They probably help the receptors for the relieving drugs to recover.

Steroids are commonly delivered from brown, red or orange coloured **inhalers**. In this form they are taken every day, usually twice a day, not to reverse an attack but to reduce the likelihood of an attack taking place. The build-up in this vital preventive role is slow: it may take a week or a fortnight, and this must be allowed for when the treatment is begun. It follows that the daily dosage should be maintained even when there are no symptoms; after all, a lack of symptoms is what the treatment aims to achieve.

The inhaled steroids do not provide a *cure* for asthma. This means that many patients stay on preventive treatment for life. In children, who may grow out of asthma, the treatment is reviewed after, say, a year. If peak flow readings (described in Chapter Seven) show that episodes of breathlessness have become rare, then the preventive treatment may be stopped for a trial period.

Using inhaled steroids safely

When first introduced, cortico-steroids were given (as tablets) in large doses to treat rheumatoid arthritis on a continuous basis, and many unpleasant side-effects resulted (see page 105). Athletes sometimes use *anabolic steroids* to build muscle mass. These are

approved name	brand names widely used in U.K.	range of doses in µg. per puff
beclomethasone dipproprionate	Aerobec	50–250
	Becodisk	100–400
	Becotide	50–200
	Becloforte	250
	Diskhaler	400
	Filair	50–250
	Rotacaps	100–400
fluticasone propionate	Flixotide Diskhaler	50–250
budesonide	Pulmicort	50–200
	Turbohaler	100–400

This table shows that most brands are available in a range of strengths. 1 mg. = 1,000 µg. (micrograms).

Steroids are also given as tablets. I have preferred to deal with this in a separate section under the heading 'acute savers', on page 104.

quite different from the *cortico-steroids*, which have no body-building potential.

With today's inhaled steroids side-effects are uncommon. This is because the drug is delivered directly to where it is needed, to the tiny air passages, so the amount is very small. A few people develop a fungal infection in the throat (*candida* or 'thrush') which is recognized when white spots appear in the mouth. This can usually be avoided by rinsing the mouth after inhaling, and by using a spacer. If that fails, there are special lozenges to treat the spots, or natural live yogurt can be taken daily.

A small minority of patients have severe asthma which requires very high doses of inhaled steroid (over 2,000 micrograms a

Some common brand names: inhaled steroids

	U.K.	U.S.A.	Canada	Australia	New Zealand
beclomethasone diproprionate					
Aerobec	√	×	×	×	*Respocort*
Becodisk	√	×	√	×	√
Becotide	√	×	×	√	√
Becloforte	√			√	
Beclovent	×	√	√	×	×
Vanceril	×	√	√	×	×
Filair	√				
fluticasone propionate					
Flixotide Diskhaler	√	×	×	×	×
budesonide					
Pulmicort	√	×	√	√	√

In the U.S.A. and Canada, other inhaled steroids include triamcinalone acetonide (Azmacort) and flunisolide (Bronzalide and AeroBid).

√ listed in 1993
× not listed in 1993

day). As explained, 70–90 per cent of an inhaled drug is swallowed. To avoid side-effects, the inhaled steroids are designed to be poorly absorbed from the intestine and to be rapidly broken down in the liver and so become harmless. They are said to achieve a low 'bio-availability'. This is true of Pulmicort and also of the new fluticasone propionate (Flixotide), which has a bio-availability close to zero.

Inhaled steroids are usually taken twice a day, preferably in the morning before breakfast and in the evening before retiring. They work only if they are taken *regularly*. They start to take effect in a few days but may require several weeks to heal the airways and rid them of inflammation. They are *preventers* and as such are taken even when there are no symptoms. If you take them before brushing your teeth, you can wash out any drug remaining in the mouth, and are unlikely to forget!

There are many different kinds of inhaler devices. The pros and cons of these will be discussed in the next chapter.

c2 Non-steroidal anti-inflammatory ⊗

(a) Sodium cromoglycate: Cromolyn/Intal

The name 'Intal' is shorthand for 'interferes with allergy', but in the *International Consensus Report on the Treatment of Asthma* it is referred to as an 'anti-inflammatory, non-steroid preventer'. It is known as Cromolyn in the USA. It acts by stabilizing the mast cells and probably also inhibits many of the inflammatory cells, including macrophages, neutrophils and eosinophils, including those responsible for the second-phase attack. Like the other preventers, it will not reverse spasm of the airway muscles. However, if given *before* exposure to an allergen such as pollen or house dust, it can in many people prevent symptoms. It can be used in conjunction with inhaled steroids.

Intal may, on its own, take 4–6 weeks to reduce inflammation, though an effect on symptoms may be seen before this time, and parents and children should persevere! Intal's great advantage is that it has an excellent safety record. Some people get a dry throat, but this can be relieved with a glass of water. It is therefore recommended in the Consensus Guidelines (see page 129) as the first-line treatment for asthma in children, especially as allergic asthma is common in young people. Intal is also used as an extra dose before exercise; it should be taken an hour beforehand.

In the U.S.A. Intal has become established as a replacement for theophylline, having similar therapeutic benefit but without theophylline's side-effects. It is not confined to children; adults with severe and persistent asthma, including 'second-phase' attacks, have been shown to benefit.

Intal is taken either as a powder from a capsule (Spincap) dispensed by a 'Spinhaler' or as a metered dose from an aerosol inhaler, or by using a nebulizer when a child cannot manage the other methods. A recent introduction, Fisonair, is an inhaler with a spacer, for children who cannot use the standard aerosol inhaler.

How Intal was discovered

The late Dr Roger Altounyan was employed by a drug company to organize trials of compounds related to 'khellin'. This was the active part of a plant, Ammi visnage, used in biblical times as a bronchodilator. Dr Altounyan distrusted animal experiments, believing that 'the only thing a guinea pig has in common with man is that neither wags a tail'; he tested the compounds on himself, a severe asthmatic. After many discouraging trials he realized that he should be testing it not as a bronchodilator (for which purpose Intal proved ineffective) but as a shield against allergic asthma.

The second problem was to discover a means of delivering the drug in a large enough dose straight to the airways. Dr Altounyan recalled his war years sitting behind the propeller at the controls of a Spitfire fighter; he then developed the Spinhaler, which enables the patient to draw in the powder by a sharp intake of breath.

Nowadays it can cost up to £50 million to develop and test a new drug before it is released for general use. No fewer than sixty drug companies have tried to find a compound with properties similar to those of Intal, and all apart from Fisons have failed. This helps to explain why radically new breakthroughs in drug treatment are rare and why improvements mainly take the form of better administration rather than radically new discoveries.

(b) Aerocrom

It is difficult to remember to take a medicine four times a day. However, by combining in one preparation 1mg. of sodium cromoglycate with a reliever (100mg. of salbutamol), it is more likely to be taken as a regular dose. This new compound is called Aerocrom and it is taken as two puffs four times each day, not on an 'as-needed' basis. It is not at present licensed for use by children under twelve years of age.

(c) Nedocromil sodium (Tilade)

Like Intal, this has been developed as a 'first-step' anti-inflammatory agent which does not contain steroids. It has a similar profile to that of Intal but probably has a stronger action against inflammation and the late-phase response. Like Intal, it is not designed to relieve an attack but to prevent attacks by regular daily use. It is likely to be especially useful in treating adults with allergic asthma which is mild to moderately severe, and (especially in the USA) to replace sustained-release theophyllines. Steroids can be used in addition.

The mode of action is similar to that of Intal and there are no significant side-effects. The main ones (headache and stomach upsets) are mild and soon pass. It is delivered from a metered-dose pressurized inhaler, taken as two puffs four times daily, reducing to two puffs twice daily. A spacing device ('Tilade Mint Syncroner') is now available and this helps you to check your inhaler technique.

Anti-allergic ⊗

C3 anti-histamine

Ketotifen (Zaditen) is a preventive medicine which is much prescribed on the continent of Europe. It is aimed mainly at mild allergic asthma in children. It is taken as a syrup or as tablets, which are easy for children to use. However, it is much less effective than the other preventers; it may take months to show benefit and, being an anti-histamine, is likely to cause drowsiness.

Group D: **Acute savers †**

In a very severe attack the patient or doctor needs a more powerful remedy than those we have considered so far. As far as the patient is concerned, he or she can be provided with a 'crisis plan' which is based on:

- a high dose of steroid tablets (prednisolone) sustained over 7–10 days
- plus a high dose of relieving medicine (a bronchodilator such as Ventolin or Bricanyl) taken from a large canister spacer. The equivalent of 30 or 40 puffs may be needed. As an alternative, it may be taken from a nebulizer, over ten minutes.

Steroid tablets

Steroids can be taken as tablets by what is confusingly known as the 'oral route'. This means that the drug enters the general circulation before it reaches the airways. This can be used for *prevention*:

- at the full dose and on a regular basis to maintain control when the asthma is persistent and severe and all other methods have failed (this is uncommon)
- to respond with a low dose to a more than usually severe challenge to the airways, such as the onset of a head cold, or exposure to severe weather or to allergens not normally encountered, in advance of any worsening of the asthma. An alternative is to increase the dosage of the inhaled steroid for the duration of the challenge, but with some patients this may not be sufficient

Tablet steroids can also provide *relief* and be used:

- to damp down inflammation at the full dose when the asthma is out of control and the other relievers have failed, in accordance with a 'crisis plan' agreed in advance with the doctor. A full effect is achieved in six hours.

The aim in these procedures is to reduce the number of inflammatory cells which arrive in the airway tissues by modifying cell reactions in the bloodstream. The way this works is not known for certain, but one suggestion is described on page 32. There is also a reduction in the output of mucus (phlegm).

The steroids used are prednisone and prednisolone, which are similar. There are various brand names which mostly manage to start with Pred-, but which also include Decortisyl, Betmelan etc. There is a soluble form called Prednesol, which is useful for children, and an enteric-coated form (Deltacortril) which reduces the risk of indigestion and ulcers associated with steroids.

The dose of tablet steroid depends on age and the severity of the attack. In an adult the *full* dose is likely to be between six and eight 5 mg. tablets a day, and four to six tablets for a child. To relieve an attack, the treatment is continued for a week to a fortnight, reduced daily down to zero and replaced with an inhaled steroid (or Intal). (mg. is short for 'milligram', one-thousandth part of a gram).

Steroids are also given by injection when the doctor is faced with a severe attack. This is usually followed by a course of Prednisolone tablets, which ends with a decreasing dosage and is then replaced with inhaled steroids to provide daily maintenance.

The safety of steroid tablets

Three or four short courses of steroid tablets in the space of a year are not likely to cause any of the side-effects which a high dose sustained over many months might incur. The *possible* side-effects of such a sustained course include a gain in weight, especially in the face and body. There can more rarely be a loss of bone density, and this will be most likely to affect people with osteoporosis. There is a heightened risk of diabetes in those who are prone to it, and of cataracts.

There is another risk when prednisone or prednisolone are given at a level which *exceeds* 5 mg. daily for more than a few months. This will tend to make the body's own steroid-producing glands (the adrenals) lazy, so that they are not able to respond when the body needs more steroids to cope with the stress of an emergency, for example an operation or illness, or an accident. Asthmatics on continuous tablet steroids should carry a bracelet obtainable from Medic-Alert, to warn doctors to give *extra* steroids in an emergency.

Other medicines

Medicines in combination

Doctors do not usually approve of a formulation in which *preventers* and *relievers* are combined so that the relative doses are fixed in advance. Some specialists would argue that that means taking extra doses of relievers which are not needed. Examples are

Aerocrom: This is described on page 103.

Duovent: This is a combination of a selective reliever (fenoterol) and ipratropium. The idea is that the two bronchodilators in combination will be more effective in certain kinds of asthma than either used on its own.

Franol: I used to help to market this brand and did so by arranging demonstrations of breathing exercises up and down the country conducted by cheerful physiotherapists. It is a tablet which contains ephedrine and theophylline, non-selective relievers which can stimulate the heart muscles. Ephedrine is unsuitable for the elderly becaue it can affect bladder opening adversely.

Ventide: By combining salbutamol (a reliever) with beclomethasone (a preventer) in Rotacaps, it is hoped that absent-minded people will remember to take both!

Medicines that are not appropriate

Patients receive bad as well as good advice and may be under the temptation to search in their medicine cupboards for a remedy without realizing that a specialist would consider it to be inappropriate.

Antihistamines no longer produce drowsiness. However, all they do is counteract histamine. In asthma this is only one of the many mediators which contribute to the attacks.

Cough mixtures are designed to decrease the cough reflex and are based on codeine. They will not relieve an asthmatic cough. They tend to make the phlegm sticky and harder to remove. To treat night cough in children, see page 182.

Mucolytics are designed to help cough up mucus. They do not work in asthma. If there is a copious discharge of mucus, this probably means that inhaled steroids should be used to damp down the discharge from the mucus glands.

Sleeping tablets may seem to be a good idea when there is asthma at night. They are definitely not suitable when the patient is liable to severe attacks, because every ounce of energy is needed to keep on forcing the breath in and out of the lungs. Even in mild asthma, sleeping tablets may be dangerous because it can be hard to predict whether the asthma will remain mild.

Are antibiotics a suitable treatment?

If a sample of patients was asked whether they find that antibiotics help them to control their asthma, most would reply that they believe they are of benefit; and many GPs prescribe antibiotics for asthmatics. The antibiotic most commonly prescribed is amoxycillin, a capsule to be taken three times a day for a full course of ten days. Any shorter course might encourage resistant bacteria to flourish.

The scientists mostly take a different view. They agree that attacks of asthma may be triggered by head colds, sore throats and (less commonly) influenza. But these infections are mainly due to viruses, and antibiotics are powerless against viruses, so there is no point in prescribing them. Furthermore the production of phlegm in asthma, however copious, does not necessarily mean that there is a chest infection. The asthma is mimicking an infection and the phlegm usually consists not of viruses or bacteria but of mucus and dead cells resulting from the inflammation.

Why then do so many patients with persistent asthma believe that antibiotics can help reduce the severity or frequency of the asthma? Are they simply deluded? One reason is that in older people the asthma is often mixed with a bronchitic infection, and it is hard to separate them from each other. Another reason is that viruses can be followed by 'secondary invaders'; these are bacteria which can descend to the chest and which can be overwhelmed by a course of antibiotics. Recent research seems to support this view. This has shown that invading bacteria can damage the linings of the air passages and expose the nerves which lie beneath them so that they react to the irritants which arrive with each breath. The bacteria may also set in train the inflammatory response.

However, the new technique of 'lavage', collecting mucus from asthmatic airways by washing it away, using volunteers, has revealed that bacteria are rarely found in the mucus. It follows that antibiotics are generally unnecessary, especially in childhood asthma. When they are prescribed, they are used in addition to the bronchodilators and steroids and not as a substitute for them.

The role of oxygen

When an acutely ill asthmatic is admitted to hospital, oxygen is likely to be given, since the level of oxygen in the blood is likely to be low. Oxygen is often given by the ambulance crew who take the patient to hospital – and a great relief this is, as I can testify. Should oxygen be kept in the home? Physicians do not usually recommend this; it may be used excessively so that a patient comes to depend on it.

As explained on page 37, there are related lung disorders (emphysema and chronic bronchitis) which may require the use of an oxygen concentrator in the home.

Current attitudes to treatment

In 1993, a Gallup survey was carried out in the UK for a pharmaceutical company which discovered that attitudes to taking medicines are still lagging some way behind current medical opinion. I hope that any reader who has travelled thus far with me will have an informed view on the opinions expressed.

A: 'I don't like to feel my body has to rely on treatment' 75 per cent

B: 'I am more likely to use a reliever than a preventer' 58 per cent

C: 'The fewer side-effects from the medicines, the better I feel' 51 per cent

D: 'I prefer to take a preventer only as needed' 46 per cent

E: 'I don't need a preventer; my reliever makes me feel better' 31 per cent

F: 'My inhaler makes me feel my asthma is worse' 39 per cent

We would all agree with (A) and (C) but accept that treatment (and some side-effects) may be inevitable. I hope my readers will disagree with (B), (D) and (if the reliever is used more than three times a week) with (E). It may, of course, be the case that the 31 per cent had only mild asthma. (F) suggests that the wrong kind of inhaler has been used or has been used incorrectly.

The search for new medicines

Scientists in many countries are trying to find new ways of blocking the immune response in the airways, without suppressing the body's immune sytem in a general way.

Cyclosporin is a powerful anti-inflammatory agent which is used both after transplant surgery and to treat people with cancer. It has been used successfully to help people whose asthma does not respond to steroids. Unfortunately, it acts on the body's immune sytem and so reduces its defences against infections; in addition it has many unpleasant side-effects. The prospect for the future is that newer and safer forms may be developed from it.

Drugs, such as cromakalim, are being investigated which could make the airway muscles less twitchy by reducing the vagus nerves' response (see page 95). Drugs are being tested which would frustrate the white cells such as leukotrienes which invade the airways.

As more is known about the way existing drugs act to reduce the symptoms of asthma, so it may be possible to modify them, either to reduce any side-effects or to make them even more effective.

CHAPTER FIVE

A Closer Look at the Inhalers

Introduction

Since asthma is mostly triggered when people inhale allergens or irritants, it is not surprising that inhalation is also the best way of delivering the medicines used as the first line of defence. When taken by the inhaled route, the medicine is directed straight to where it is required: the air passages. This means that only a tiny dose is needed to achieve its purpose and, as a result, side-effects are reduced to a minimum. Not all the spray reaches the airways, but the part which is swallowed is itself so small that it causes no upsets unless the patient is extremely sensitive to the particular drug or is using the device far too often.

In the comparatively rare case in which most of the airways are so badly plugged with mucus that the spray cannot reach them, then the medicine has to be taken by way of a tablet or syrup. In a very severe attack an injection may be needed.

There are three ways in which a medicine can be inhaled:

as an aerosol spray	**as a dry powder**	**as a solution**
(bulb inhaler)	Spinhaler	nebulizer
metered-dose inhaler	Rotahaler	
pressurized inhaler plus spacer	Diskhaler Turbohaler	
Autohaler		

The Brovon bulb inhaler is still available but is no longer widely used. I have included it because it illustrates how a drug in solution can be turned into a fine spray. When it was introduced in the 1930s it was a great advance because until then patients were given either ephedrine as a tablet, resulting in nervous agitation, or adrenaline by injection by a doctor. By squeezing the bulb, a jet of air could be passed over a thin tube and so draw up the medicine in solution and at the same time produce a vapour, in much the same way that a carburettor in a car produces petrol vapour. The disadvantages were that the glass tubes became blocked, the dose varied with the squeeze and many droplets were probably too large to reach the smaller airways.

Metered-dose aerosol inhalers

The aim is to produce a single measured dose in the form of a fine spray. The medicine is suspended in a liquid propellant (freon) inside a pressurized container. When the valve is opened, the propellant forces the mixture out at great speed, emerging as a cloud of fine particles which hit the back of the throat. At this stage the mixture is made up of propellant, lubricant and a small proportion of medicine. The metering chamber then refills in about thirty seconds and the inhaler is ready for a second puff. The freon gas is used because of its safety. A small minority of asthmatics can be irritated by the gas and the carriers; this can cause spasm, but is immediately reversed if it is a bronchodilator which is being delivered. (Some people are worried that aerosols containing C.F.C.s – chlorinated hydrocarbons – are making holes in the earth's ozone layer and letting in a dangerous amount of ultra-violet light. Some kinds of medical aerosols may in due course be banned, but it is to be hoped that they will be replaced by more acceptable propellants. If you are concerned about this problem, you can use a dry powder inhaler instead.)

Metered-dose aerosol inhalers may be said to have transformed

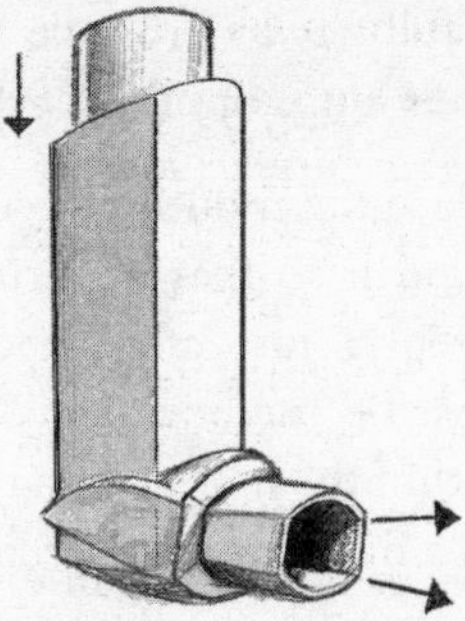

Fig. 9. Metered-dose aerosol inhaler

the treatment of asthma since the first one, the 'Medihaler', was introduced in the mid-1960s. The aerosol form is used to deliver not only the *relievers* (Ventolin, Bricanyl and Berotec) but also the *preventers* (Becotide, Filair, Pulmicort and Intal) and a *protector* (Serevent). They are convenient, carry 100 to 200 doses and account for the majority of prescriptions written for asthma. Allen & Hanburys supply a Haleraid grip for people with arthritic fingers.

The disadvantage is that an effective dose is delivered only when the device is used properly. This not only requires a good co-ordination between squeezing and breathing but it is also a performance which modest people with asthma are understandably reluctant to display in public (or in the company of friends). Always make sure that the way *you* use the inhaler has been checked by a doctor or nurse, bearing in mind that half the patients use their 'press-and-breathe' inhalers incorrectly; after fresh teaching, half revert quite soon to the incorrect way.

1 It is best to use the inhaler standing up, with the head tipped back slightly.

2 Remove the cover and shake the inhaler vigorously in order to mix the medicine with the propellant.

3 Holding the inhaler between thumb and forefinger, breathe out gently, not so fully as to provoke a cough but with the aim of emptying your lungs of most of the air you feel inside them.

4 Immediately place the mouthpiece in the mouth and close the lips tightly round it so that no drug escapes. Start to inhale, slowly and deeply; just after you have started, press the canister quite hard – use both hands if necessary. This is done by squeezing thumb and forefinger together. Continue to breathe in until a full breath has been taken.

5 Hold your breath for about ten seconds, or as long as is comfortable, to make sure you do not expel the medicine you have just taken in.

6 Before taking a second puff, allow half a minute to pass before squeezing again. This will give the metering chamber time to refill.

7 Replace the cap on the mouthpiece.

It is not easy to remember the names of the medicines, especially when short of breath or in the early hours of the morning. The colours on the plastic actuator case help: it is worth remembering that Ventolin is blue, Becotide 50 is light beige, Becotide 100 is brown and Becloforte a maroon red. Serevent is turquoise. These colours can be hard to see in a low light, so I cut a nick in the mouthpiece of the blue inhaler since this is the one needed to relieve breathlessness as it occurs.

All too often the inhaler is found to be out of action, either because it has been mislaid or because it is empty. At night, when needed to relieve the 3 a.m. 'morning dip', it seems to have disappeared into the bedclothes. During the day, a quick change of clothes may result in leaving home without it. Old hands at this game make sure that they practise good housekeeping, checking each week where the inhalers are and ensuring that they are well charged. I use a letter-weighing scale to tell me just how much solution remains inside. Another trick is to remove

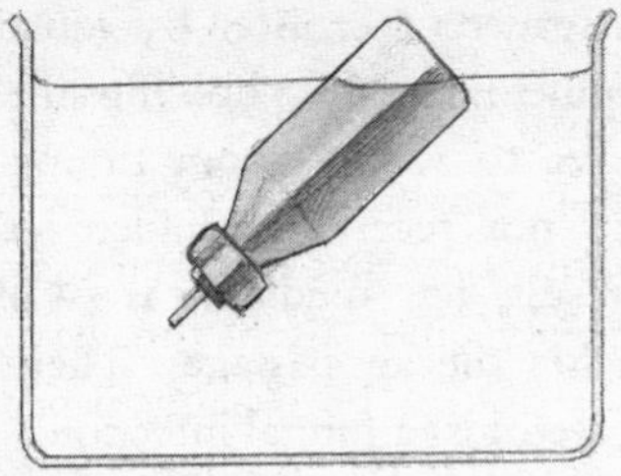

Fig. 10. One-quarter full

the metal canister and place it in water: if it sinks, it is full; if it floats flat, it is empty; and if it rests suspended at an angle, then it is one-quarter full. It is prudent to leave inhalers in a number of places: in the briefcase or overnight bag; in the glove compartment of the car or in a drawer at the office. Some doctors initially prescribe half a dozen inhalers for this reason. They are best kept at room temperature before use. Empty inhalers should be thrown away and replenishments obtained in good time. At night, the inhaler can be placed on the bedside table or attached to the bedpost by a loop of string passed through it.

Spacers

Trials have shown that only a minority of patients use aerosol inhalers correctly. Most people forget to shake the container, or they do not breathe out before firing, or do not hold the breath after firing, or they take the second dose too soon.

Co-ordination between squeeze and breathe is not needed when **spacers** are fixed to the inhaler. The Spacer Inhaler receives the aerosol spray in a small collapsible sleeve (Bricanyl or Pulmicort). There is also a large-volume plastic canister in two designs: the **Nebuhaler** is used with Bricanyl and the **Volumatic** with Ventolin, but the metal parts of the inhaler are interchangeable. Intal can be used with a **Fisonair** spacer.

You fill the spacer or canister by squeezing the inhaler and then breathe quite normally, holding the spacer horizontally. You do not have to worry about timing, and with the large canister you do not receive a sudden jet of medicine in the mouth. As a result, less medicine is swallowed and a greater proportion reaches the air passages. There is less risk of a dry throat or (with steroids) a fungal infection.

The large-volume spacers allow time for the aerosol propellant to evaporate away from the tiny particles of the drug; this makes them small enough to penetrate into the smallest airways. Use one dose from the aerosol at a time; do not fill the container with multiple doses. The dose can be repeated many times when trying to control a severe attack with a reliever. Remember to shake before squeezing.

The large canisters are too big to carry around but can be used for night and morning doses. The **Aerochamber** is a smaller version. All spacers and canisters except the Aerochamber (described below) can be obtained on prescription. The Nebuhaler and the Volumatic can also be bought from the chemist for under £10 (ask your retail pharmacist).

Spacers and young children

Children can use a spacer on their own from three years of age upwards, having been taught how to use it when empty. The valve makes a little noise which appeals to them. If the child is under three years old, a mask (as supplied free with a Nebuhaler and known as the 'McCarthy mask') can be fitted to the spacer. The end of the spacer is tipped up to keep the valve open and the child breathes normally. For use with young children, the Medic-Aid Aerochamber with a soft mask is particularly suitable (see page 174 and Useful Addresses). If the child resists treatment, the spacer can be used when he or she is asleep. It can be decorated with stickers and introduced as a toy.

It is possible to make a spacer by inserting any aerosol inhaler

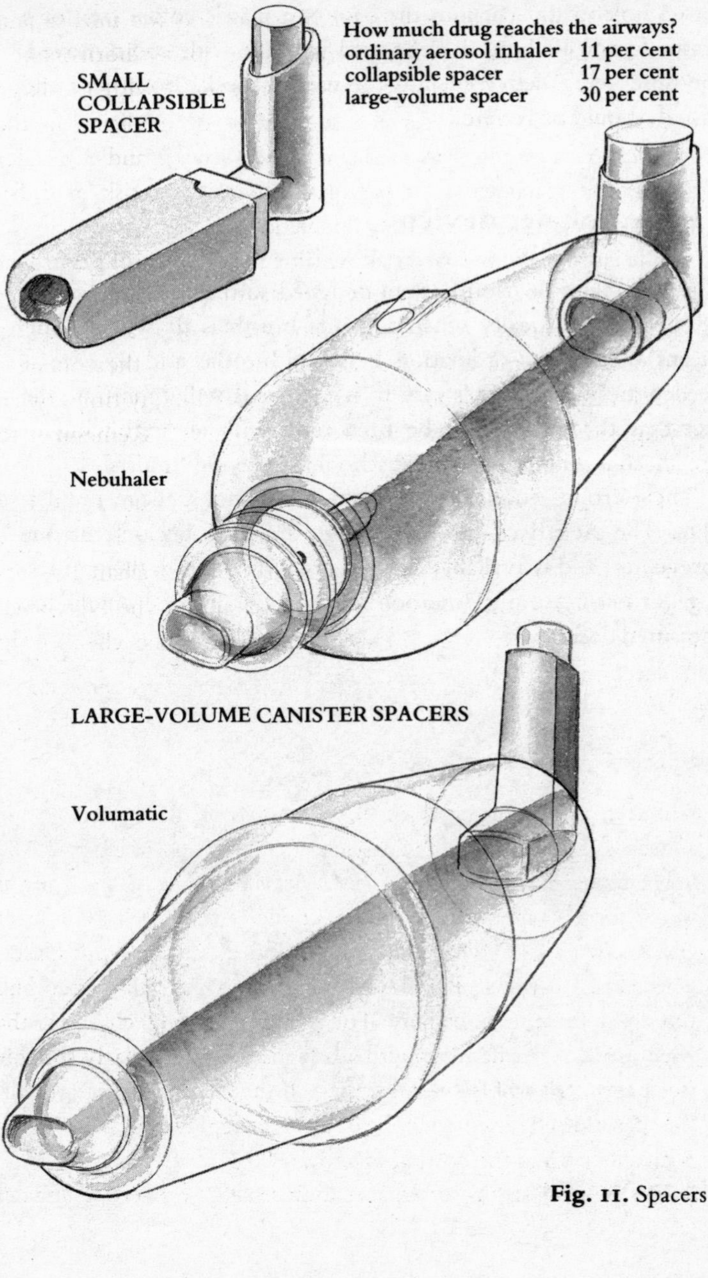
How much drug reaches the airways?
ordinary aerosol inhaler 11 per cent
collapsible spacer 17 per cent
large-volume spacer 30 per cent
SMALL COLLAPSIBLE SPACER
Nebuhaler
LARGE-VOLUME CANISTER SPACERS
Volumatic

Fig. 11. Spacers

into a hole neatly cut into the base of a plastic coffee cup; or a plastic lemonade bottle can be used with the wide end removed, the dose being delivered into the narrow neck. Both nose and mouth should be covered.

The Autohaler device

The Autohaler device has been designed so that the medicine is released automatically when a gentle breath is drawn in. This means that no co-ordination between breathe and squeeze is needed and the device is easy to use. Parents will appreciate the fact that the inhaler can be fired only with an indrawing of breath, so it will not be used at school for playing 'squirts'.

The Aerolin Autohaler dispenses salbutamol (reliever) and is blue. The AeroBec Autohaler range dispenses beclomethasone (preventer) and is available in three strengths: 50 mg. (beige); 100 mg. (brown); 250 mg. (maroon red). All the devices contain 200 measured doses.

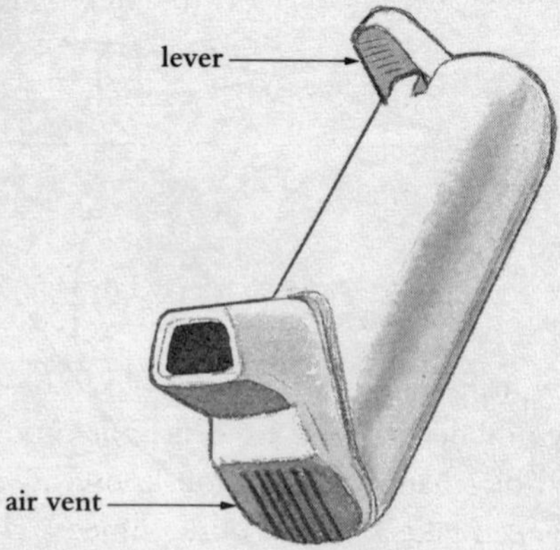

Fig. 12. Autohaler

Instructions on how to use the Autohaler are given in an information leaflet supplied with each pack:

- remove the cap and shake to mix the contents
- push the lever up; breathe out gently
- close your lips round the mouthpiece, keeping the air vent open
- breathe in steadily; when the inhaler clicks, it releases the drug. Continue to take a deep breath
- hold the breath for about ten seconds
- push the lever down to re-set the device

Dry powder inhalers

In these inhalers the medicine is in the form of a powder which is delivered when there is a sharp in-drawing of breath. In the older versions, insert a capsule (Rotacap) containing the powder into the inhaler (Rotahaler) then puncture the capsule by twisting or squeezing the device. This releases the powder and you breathe inwards without any need for co-ordination. The Intal Spinhaler is so called because it incorporates a propeller which increases the turbulence needed to separate the particles.

	Spinhaler	**Rotahaler**
sodium cromoglycate	Intal	—
salbutamol	—	Ventolin
beclomethasone	—	Becotide

Compared with the aerosol pressurized inhalers there are advantages: dry powder inhalers are easier for children and older people with arthritic hands to use; you know how many doses remain; and you can take a second dose immediately. An advantage with children is that these inhalers do not lend themselves to playing 'squirts' at school! A disadvantage of the single-dose

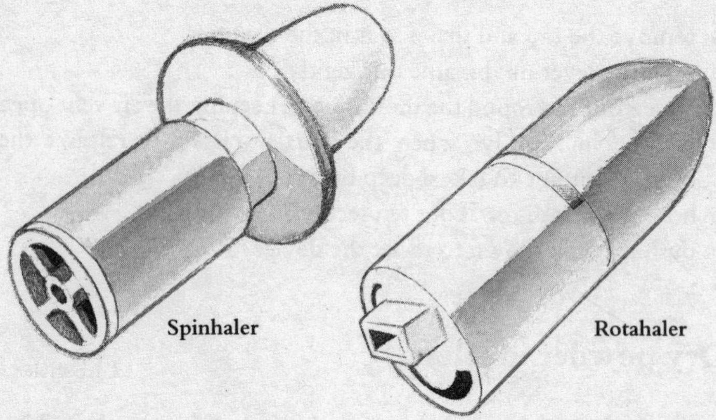

Fig. 13. Dry powder inhalers

powder inhalers is that they have to be reloaded each time they are used.

Multi-dose inhalers

The Diskhaler dispenses Ventolin, Becotide, Flixotide or Serevent as a dry powder from a disk which contains eight blisters, each containing a single dose. This makes it easy to check how many doses have been taken. When all eight doses have been discharged, a new disk is fitted. There is a lactose carrier, the taste of which confirms that the drug has been delivered.

The Turbohaler uses a rotating scoop. When twisted, this collects a tiny amount of drug from a reservoir. The drug is drawn upwards through spiral tubes which disperse the particles, the motive power being a sharp indrawing of breath. Unlike all other inhalers (powder or aerosol), there are no carriers to act as irritants, and this also means that 200 doses can be stored in a space inside the device which is no larger than a capsule. The Turbohaler can dispense Bricanyl (a reliever) or Pulmicort (a

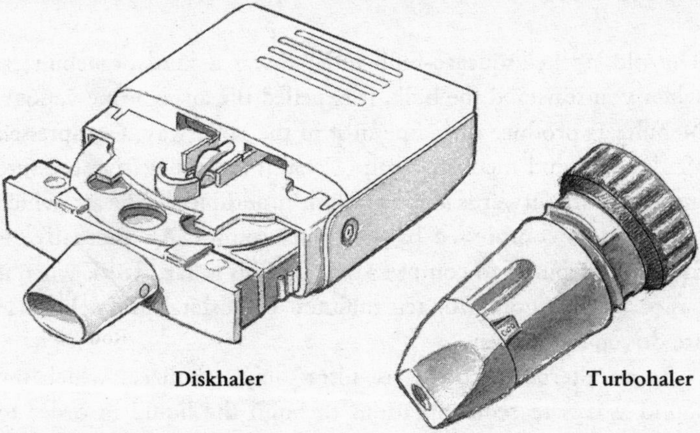

Fig. 14. Multi-dose inhalers

preventer). Clinical trials have shown that most patients can use the inhaler even when the asthma is severe. The only drawbacks are that there is no noise or taste to convince you that the medicine has been taken, and it is difficult to tell how many doses remain in the device. A special grip can be fitted to help people with arthritic fingers: consult your retail pharmacist.

	Diskhaler	**Turbohaler**	**Autohaler**
reliever			
salbutamol	Ventodisk		Aerolin
terbutaline		Bricanyl	
preventer			
beclomethasone	Becodisk		Aerobec
budesonide		Pulmicort	
fluticasone	Flixotide		
protector			
salmeterol	Serevent		

Nebulizers

The old pocket squeeze-bulb inhaler was a kind of nebulizer: when you squeezed the bulb, it expelled the air as a fine vapour. Nebulizers produce their fine mist in the same way. Compressed air draws liquid medicine from a chamber by negative pressure upwards and outwards into a mask or mouthpiece. The air, which is filtered, is compressed by an electric pump. An alternative is to use a footpump to compress the air. This is hard work when it has to be kept going for ten minutes. In hospitals the nebulizers are driven by oxygen.

As an alternative there are ultra-sonic nebulizers which use sound waves to send vibrations through the liquid in order to form the vapour. They have the advantage of being silent and the disadvantage of being even more expensive than the compressed-air machines.

Which drugs can be nebulized?

Most of the drugs in common use can be nebulized, with the exception of the theophyllines. The drugs are provided in solution in small bottles or ampoules. Among the relievers Ventolin, Bricanyl, Berotec and Atrovent can be delivered by nebulizer. Among the preventers Intal, Becotide and Pulmicort can be administered in this way. However, the *protectors* are not at present nebulized.

Ventolin, Bricanyl and Intal are available as single-dose ampoules; multi-dose bottles are available for Ventolin, Bricanyl, Atrovent and Becotide, but not for Intal.

Advantages and disadvantages

A device which is complicated, expensive (£130–180) and which makes an impressive noise has an aura of magic about it. Yet it

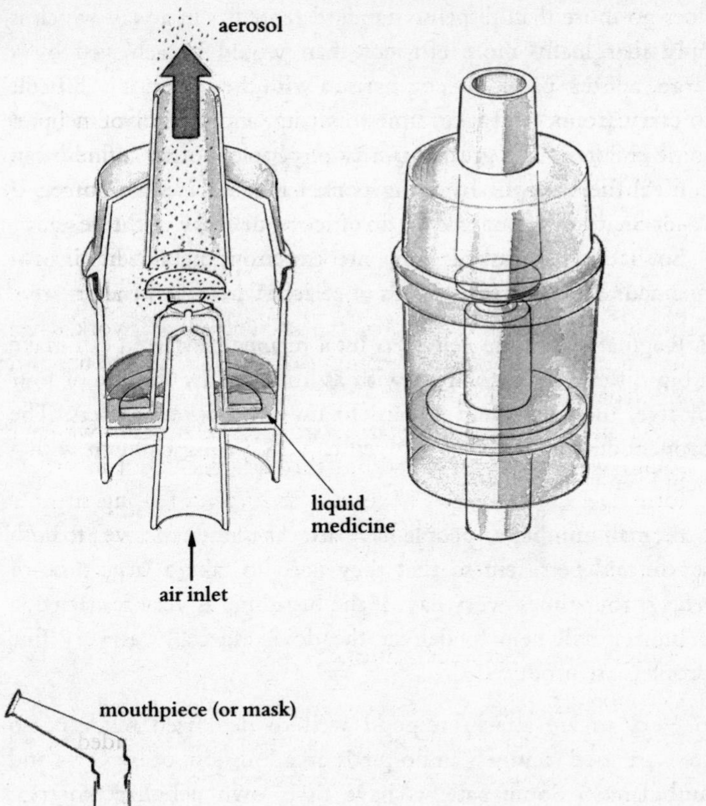

Fig. 15. The way a nebulizer works

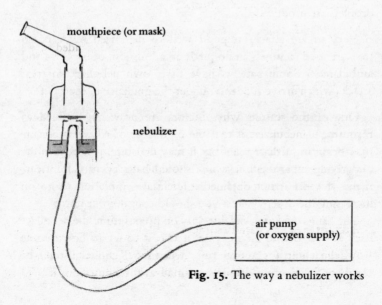

does no more than dispense standard remedies in a way which is only marginally more efficient than would be achieved by a large canister spacer. By comparison with the spacer, it is difficult to carry around and takes time to set up, and the noise can upset some children. The great majority of people, young and old, can control their asthma by using pocket inhalers (with a spacer, if co-ordination is poor and for an efficient delivery of the dose).

So, it may be asked, why are expensive nebulizers recommended? There are three kinds of patient who may benefit:

- Regular use of the *preventers* Intal or inhaled steroid can make a big difference to children with asthma. Below the age of four or five, they may find it hard to use the pocket inhalers. The bronchodilator Atrovent is given to very young children with a nebulizer
- A small number of people have attacks of asthma that are both severe and persistent so that they need to take a large dose of *reliever* four times every day. If the breathing is very restricted, a nebulizer will help to deliver the dose, especially as very fine droplets are produced
- Very severe attacks respond well to nebulized relievers, so they are used routinely in hospitals on admission, or by G.P.s and ambulances. Some patients have their own nebulizer to treat attacks which arrive suddenly, under the guidance of their G.P.

One of the reasons why doctors are now less inclined to recommend nebulizers is that the high dose of *reliever* medicine may bring immediate relief but it may do nothing to reduce the underlying inflammation which should have priority for treatment. If relief is not obtained, there is a temptation to go on increasing the dose, whereas you should consult your doctor.

The drugs used are available only on prescription; the nebulizer itself is not. Before buying one, it is best to try to borrow one from the clinic for a trial run. The model chosen should be capable of delivering droplets as small as three microns. If used each day, a record of 'peak flow' should be kept, as explained in the next chapter. Bacteria flourish in the nebulizing chamber so it should be kept clean at all times. The air pump should be serviced twice a year; I understand that some hospitals have a home nebulizer service for this purpose.

If the asthma is severe enough to need a nebulizer, then you should keep a check on the asthma with a peak flow meter, as explained in Chapter Six.

Are there side-effects?

With preventive medicines they are rare, and Intal has no serious side-effects. With the nebulized *relievers* there can be dangers. Trembling of the hands is not serious, but a rapid or irregular heartbeat is possible, and care has to be taken with elderly patients whose heart is already affected in some way.

CHAPTER SIX

Adjusting the Treatment

How bad is the asthma?

Picture the consultation – not as the patient but as the doctor! Each patient has a different story to tell, in language far removed from the precise terms of medical science. 'Would you say that the attacks are mild or severe?' One will describe as mild symptoms which another will consider to be severe. Some agreed definitions are needed.

In their research programme, Fisons Pharmaceuticals rely heavily on patients' descriptions of their asthma. They use the table below to enable patients to record the severity of their attacks. I have attached my own labels ('episodic and mild' etc.) for the purpose of this chapter.

scale		
0	no symptoms of wheeze or breathlessness	
1	occasional wheeze or breathlessness, which is easily reversed with an inhaled bronchodilator	*episodic & mild*
2	wheeziness or shortage of breath occurs most of the time but does not interfere with the usual activities at home or at work	*persistent & mild*
3	wheeziness or shortage of breath occurs most of the time and there is some interference with the usual activities	*persistent & severe*

4	asthma very bad. Could not go to school/work or carry out the usual household duties	***acute & severe***

We also need to describe the breathing difficulties which take place *at night*. In mild and persistent asthma, sleep may be interrupted several times a week but a puff from the relieving inhaler quickly restores the breathing to its usual level. In severe asthma, sleep is impossible.

In anyone with asthma, the severity may change from one season to another, or from one week to the next. In my personal recollection, asthma in childhood used to be mild – except at the height of the pollen season, when it became severe and persistent. From late middle age it became persistent, with no remission, and is especially likely to be severe when the weather is cold or unsettled.

Patients with persistent asthma are particularly at risk that their asthma may deteriorate into a very severe attack. This is described on page 138.

Measuring 'peak flow'

People with asthma often think they know just how bad their asthma is by the feeling of tightness in their chest. Research in Australia has demonstrated that this can be misleading. Some mornings, when I wake, the asthma may seem severe but then subside after a single puff from the relieving inhaler. A few days later it may appear to be mild, until I begin to stir – and then I find I am very short of breath. When resting, only a little oxygen is required and an absence of wheeze or breathlessness does not mean that the airways are free from obstruction.

What is needed is some objective way of measuring lung capacity using a scale of severity. This is now possible by using a simple peak flow meter, which will be described fully in the next chapter.

How does the doctor choose the treatments?

We have studied the illness and its many triggers. We have surveyed the remedies, including the medicines which are used nowadays, and we have looked at the various ways in which they can be taken. We then considered how the severity of the illness could be assessed by observing the symptoms and by measuring the peak flow. Peak flow readings can also be used to decide whether or not the treatment has been effective.

Let us now return to the surgery and put ourselves in the place of the doctor. How does he decide what treatment to prescribe? First of all, there must be a detailed case history. This will reveal whether the asthma is episodic (occasional) or persistent; whether it is usually mild or quite often severe. A note will be made as to whether there is wheezing or coughing at night, after exercise, or after meals. The patient may be asked to take home a peak flow meter and enter readings on a diary card, and to return to the surgery after a set time for a further assessment. The doctor may also want to know:

- what tends to provoke the attacks? The list to be ticked includes seasonal factors, animals, house dust, head colds, exercise, cold air, emotion, food, something at work
- does anyone in the family smoke? Do you smoke?
- what are the present symptoms? (Mucus? Wheeze? Cough?)
- when are the symptoms most troublesome?
- what treatments have been used? What are being used at present? How many times a day?
- do the symptoms disappear shortly after treatment, or do they fail to respond?

An allergist would probe further into the kind of triggers that the patient or parent believes are responsible for the attacks.

For how long do I need to go on taking the medicines?

The Guidelines in the next section allow for stepping down treatment as well as for stepping up. With children it is advisable to continue for a year before making a decision to stop treatment altogether, and then only if the symptoms are mild and with very few episodes of wheezing. In adults, treatment is usually for a lifetime, unless the episodes are few and far between.

The 'BTS Guidelines'

Many doctors nowadays follow a step-by-step system of treatment which was first published in 1990 in the *British Medical Journal*. This resulted from the deliberations of a committee of scientists, chest physicians, general practitioners and a patient (myself).

The Guidelines consist of a series of steps, starting with the assumption that the asthma is mild, then working through increasing degrees of severity and adjusting the treatment accordingly. They must be distinguished from the steps used by a patient when controlling his or her asthma on a daily basis in accordance with a treatment plan.

Step 1: *the asthma is mild and intermittent:* use an inhaled bronchodilator (*reliever*) as needed (e.g. Ventolin, Bricanyl, Berotec).

Step 2: *the reliever is needed more than once a day and/or there is wheeziness at night:* add a *preventer* on a daily basis: use Intal or Tilade four times a day. If this does not achieve control, use as well or instead an inhaled steroid (Becotide, Becloforte, Filair, Flixotide or Pulmicort), taken twice daily.

Step 3: *the symptoms persist:* increase the inhaled steroid to four times daily, up to a maximum of 2,000 μg., using a large-volume spacer.

Step 4: *control is still not achieved, night asthma persists:* add a short course of tablet steroid at a high dose (1 mg. per kilogram of bodyweight per day). At this stage the doctor may consider as an addition a *trial* of one or more of: a long-acting *reliever* (e.g. slow-release theophylline); or Atrovent; or a *protector* (Serevent or Bambec); or Intal or Tilade.

Step down: *after 3–6 months, the symptoms are well controlled:* move down a step in treatment, for example to inhaled steroid twice a day, with the additional treatments in Step 4 reconsidered.

Four case histories

In books I prefer to learn about medicine through case histories. The ones which follow are actual histories, with the names changed. Each one could apply, in principle, to any age group above infancy.

It should be borne in mind that, as the Guidelines suggest, all treatment is on a trial-and-error basis. Doctors vary in their approach to medication and have to take into account factors (such as home circumstances, age, experience and other illnesses) which cannot be included here.

To remind you what the treatments are aiming to achieve, the following symbols are used:

relieving drugs	a sword †	bronchodilators
protecting drugs	a shield ⊗	long-acting relievers
preventing drugs	a shield ⊗	anti-inflammatory and anti-allergic drugs

A. Mild episodic asthma

Patient: 'I just wheeze sometimes.'

Peter, a young man in his early thirties, had mild, episodic asthma as a child, but fortunately grew out of it in his teens. By the time he was in his twenties he had no symptoms of wheeze or breathlessness. He has recently become very health-conscious and keen to keep fit and avoid 'middle-age flab'. He has now cut down on animal fats, has a high-fibre diet, eats lots of fruit, fish and vegetables and has taken up marathon running. It is hard luck that, with all that sensible attention to diet, he finds that the running makes him very short of breath after about ten minutes. He asks the doctor what he should do.

Diagnosis: episodic asthma, in this case brought on by exercise. Mainly due to spasm in the breathing tubes which will be reversed with a bronchodilator reliever.

Treatment:
† take inhaled bronchodilator when needed (Ventolin or Bricanyl)
⊗ take the bronchodilator ten minutes before exercise; and keep the inhaler handy, to be used when wheezy
⊗ as an alternative, or in addition, take Intal 30 minutes before the exercise

B. Moderate persistent asthma

Parent: 'She gets asthma quite often now, at least four or five times a week. They are not severe attacks but we feel that the asthma is not being properly controlled.'

Mary, aged five, fair haired and blue eyed, is a very lively child, advanced for her age. She had eczema as an infant, but this responded well to treatment with hydrocortisone cream. When she joined a play group she tended to get short of breath when racing round the hall. Quite recently she has started to waken her parents at night with fits of coughing and a slight shortage of breath. This is causing distress to all concerned.

It is also of concern that Mary frequently has head colds, and these are invariably followed by a spell of wheeziness, again not severe but persistent.

Diagnosis: the wheeziness after exercise, the coughing at night and the wheeziness after a virus infection all add up to typical signs of asthma. The persistence of the attacks and the night asthma (confirmed by taking peak flow readings) call for regular *preventive* treatment.

Treatment:
⊗ take Intal 3–4 times a day every day, even when there are no symptoms. In adults, and in children who are not controlled on Intal, take an inhaled steroid (Becotide, Filair, Flixotide, or Pulmicort) twice a day, every day, regardless of symptoms.
† take a bronchodilator as needed and half an hour before playing or exercise, from an inhaler (Ventolin or Bricanyl)

If, in spite of this treatment, night coughing persists, then additional treatment may be needed (see 'night cough', page 182)

With young children, mothers find that a bronchodilator given as syrup is sometimes the only way they can persuade the child to take the medicine. As an alternative they give Intal from a nebulizer.

C. Acute severe asthma

'Doctor, can you come and see me. As you can hear . . . I am very . . . short of . . . breath . . . and the inhaler does not seem to be . . . having any . . . effect.'

Sarah, aged thirty-five, developed hay fever when a teenager and this coincided with the examination months of June and July. The hay fever has remained but is well controlled on a steroid nasal spray (Beconase or Flixonase), provided she remembers to start taking it before the pollen season begins.

Quite suddenly in June 1989 she started to wake at night with coughing and wheezing – not every night but three or four times a week. By August, the symptoms had disappeared. All this was bearable – but one night in July 1990 she found herself severely short of breath and, in a state of alarm, rang the doctor.

Diagnosis: an acute and severe attack. The normally mild asthma moved into a second-phase attack, and this will not always respond to a bronchodilator given from a pocket inhaler.

Treatment:

(*a*) *before the doctor arrives*

† Much depends on what is available in the home. Ideally the patient should immediately take a high dose of tablet steroids (e.g. 8 x 5 mg. tablets of Prednisolone). If a nebulizer is available, with a relieving bronchodilator, this should be used at once. As an alternative a high dose (30–40 puffs) of bronchodilator can be taken using a large-volume spacer (Ventolin or Bricanyl)

(*b*) *when the doctor comes*

† The doctor will assess the seriousness of the attack and will probably rely on a nebulized bronchodilator in a high dose

† plus steroid in a high dose, either nebulized or as tablets of Prednisolone or as an intravenous injection of hydrocortisone. If an ambulance is called, then oxygen may be given on the way to the hospital

† if you have taken theophylline, tell the doctor

(*c*) *a plan for the future*

⊗ The high dose of tablet steroid will be maintained for at least ten days, followed by inhaled steroid (Becotide, Becloforte, Filair, Flixotide or Pulmicort) to be taken night and morning

† A bronchodilator (Ventolin or Bricanyl) will be used as needed

Assessment: (1) the doctor or nurse will check your

inhaler technique. (2) a self-management plan will be worked out for the future, as discussed in the next chapter. (3) a peak flow meter will be prescribed and a diary kept and reviewed at the next consultation.

D. Severe persistent asthma

Patient: 'I seem to wheeze most of the time and asthma wakes me at night at least three times a week. At times the attacks are difficult to control with a bronchodilator.'

Anthony, aged ten, a quiet child, has had asthma and eczema since he was eighteen months old. He was referred to the outpatients department of the Paediatric Unit at the hospital and they recommended that he should have a nebulizer at home, for administering salbutamol (a bronchodilator). Rarely do 24 hours pass without wheezing and coughing, and he has had many bad nights and a lot of time away from school. In his case the triggers were all too numerous: not only the allergic triggers of pollen in the hay season, and cats, but also non-allergic triggers such as exercise, virus infections (i.e. head colds) and laughter. His mother relied on giving salbutamol (Ventolin) through the nebulizer when the attacks became really bad but did not think that anything more could be done. One evening the attack was so bad that he was brought to the surgery, with a peak flow of 80.

Diagnosis: the asthma is both severe and persistent; the breathing tubes are hyper-responsive and react to quite small triggers. This means that there is inflammation in the airways as well as muscle spasm. The peak flow is probably depressed all the time, but it may well be possible to restore it to a normal level, given the correct treatment.

Treatment:

† Steroid tablets are taken in a high dose for a limited period

(Prednisolone) and then, when the asthma is stabilized, the treatment is changed to

⊗ an inhaled steroid taken regularly, night and morning, even when there are no symptoms (e.g. Becotide, Becloforte, Filair, Flixotide or Pulmicort in accordance with a treatment plan)

⊗ Intal, or an inhaled reliever, will be used 15 minutes before exercise

† The reliever will be used as needed (Ventolin or Bricanyl)

† In addition, the doctor will provide an emergency treatment: tablets of steroid (Prednisolone) to be taken if there is a severe attack

⊗ If troublesome night asthma persists, a slow-release reliever (theophylline, or Volmax) or a *protector* (Serevent or Bambec) as an additional measure

Assessment: a peak flow meter will be prescribed and the mother will be asked to keep a diary for 2–3 weeks, and then report back to the doctor to see if the treatment needs to be adjusted

Asthma treatment cards

It is difficult, if not impossible, to remember the plan that has been agreed with the doctor, so printed folding treatment cards are often used (an example is given on page 178). The cards record not only the routine daily treatment but also what to do if there is a severe attack. They should be updated at regular intervals. In the U.K. the cards can be obtained from the National Asthma Campaign in three versions: for adults, for children and for parents to give to school teachers.

Managing brittle asthma

This is a rare form of severe asthma. In some patients the peak flow swings up and down by about 40 per cent a day. In others, in spite of long periods of good control and regular use of preventive medicine, severe attacks take place, suddenly and with very little warning. Of all groups these are most at risk.

It is not known why these patients have brittle asthma. They are mostly anxious, but this is likely to be a consequence rather than a cause. What is known is that they tend to have lower levels of immunity: fewer Ig1 antibodies circulating in the blood and available to fight infections, compared with other people.

Dr Jon Ayres of the East Birmingham Hospital (U.K.) has made a special study of this condition and has borrowed a method of treatment from the management of diabetes. The aim is to deliver small but continuous doses over 24 hours of a *reliever* medicine (Bricanyl) by means of a slowly moving syringe and a needle inserted under the skin. Doses of inhaled steroids are maintained. This sounds disagreeable, but patients who wear these pumps can lead a full life, including regular swimming.

What to do if things go wrong

The four case histories have illustrated some of the ways in which a doctor might interpret the BTS Guidelines. From your point of view, from time to time you may feel that what has been prescribed is not achieving the desired result. What follows is a check-list which is designed to help you decide what to do if things start to go wrong. It was written by a general practitioner for his patients and has been slightly changed to suit this chapter. It assumes that you are not using a peak flow meter on a regular basis.

Your wheezes get worse when you have a cold

Increase the dose of inhaled steroid (Becotide, Becloforte, Filair, Flixotide or Pulmicort) by increasing dosage to four times a day, while the cold lasts.

You wheeze when you take exercise

Use your reliever (Ventolin or Bricanyl) beforehand: an hour ahead, if you use tablets or a syrup; ten minutes, if you use an inhaler. Or take your Intal or Tilade, just beforehand.

You wheeze when you go out into the cold

Use your reliever inhaler about ten minutes before you leave the house, even if you have no symptoms while indoors.

You wheeze when out visiting . . .

because there is something at the place to which you are usually allergic. Take your reliever from an inhaler about ten minutes before you arrive and repeat as needed. Better still, if your doctor has provided you with steroid tablets (Prednisolone), take 10 mg. every day for the duration of the visit, up to ten days, having started the day before the visit. Some people will be protected if they are taking Intal or Tilade.

You often wake at night with wheezing

Consult your doctor. He will prescribe a preventer (inhaled steroid) to damp down the inflammation. If this has not worked, he will consider in addition a slow-release reliever which will last for the whole night, or a protector (e.g. Serevent or Bambec). As far as children are concerned, this is discussed in more detail on page 182.

The reliever does not act long enough

You may find that you need to use the reliever inhaler (Ventolin, Bricanyl or Berotec) more and more frequently. This is a WARNING SIGN that the asthma is becoming more severe. *If the effect of a dose (one or two puffs) lasts for three hours or less,* you should consult the doctor.

You have become a 'slow slider'

That is to say, your wheezing has been getting gradually worse over a number of days. This is discussed in the next chapter.

Depending on the severity, you will need to increase the dose of preventer (inhaled steroid) or, if you have been given a supply of steroid tablets (Prednisolone), put yourself on a short ten-day course of these. Then consult your doctor and explain that you have used up your emergency supply.

You have a sudden severe attack . . .
that is not relieved by the bronchodilator. This is when the **crisis plan** is put into action, as explained in the next section.

When you should summon help immediately

You should call the doctor as soon as you feel that an attack is slipping out of control, after taking the medicines you have been given to relieve it. Let the expert decide.

It happened that I had a severe 'second-phase' attack (the one that occurs six hours after a much milder episode) on the very day I drafted this section. I had driven into the country to stay with friends and the weather suddenly changed, bringing out autumn mould spores in the damp atmosphere. I told the doctor who attended about the book and he commented: 'Do please tell your readers that asthma can *kill* and that, in the event of an attack which they cannot control, they should observe two golden rules':

(1) Do not delay in calling your doctor, or dial 999 for an ambulance, as soon as it is clear that this is no run-of-the-mill episode.

(2) Immediately take the relieving medicine you have available, *all at once* and not in stages. That means one puff of Bricanyl or Ventolin every 10 or 15 seconds until you feel better, up to 30 or 40 puffs. *At the same time*, start a course of Prednisolone tablets (see 'Acute Savers' on page 104).

I often remind myself that, in a crisis, it is the asthma which is dangerous, not the medicine. Here are some more suggestions, which occurred to me on this particular occasion:

(3) When away from home, make sure you have your peak flow meter. A sudden drop of half below *best* level is a danger sign (to be explained in the next chapter).

(4) A large-volume spacer should also be in your suitcase; it is the best way of achieving a high dose of relieving medicine if a nebulizer is not available (see page 115). Up to 40 puffs of Ventolin or Bricanyl can be taken in an emergency, each separated by 15 seconds.

(5) A severe attack may take place when you are out of reach of a doctor, for example on a walking holiday. Make sure that your 'crisis' plan is fully worked out in advance and that you have access to the appropriate medicines. Self-management plans are discussed fully in the next chapter.

What are the danger signs?

When the doctor answers your urgent telephone call, he or she will need to decide whether to attend in person or to summon an ambulance, or both. He will need to be given an idea as to the patient's current appearance.

All patients and carers should be aware of the warning signs that asthma is out of control. If any one of these occurs, medical help should be summoned without delay:

- the inhaler has no effect after ten minutes
- breathing is in short, sharp gasps which cannot be controlled in depth or frequency. If the wheezing ceases, this is a real *danger* signal: so little air is going in that the chest has become silent
- the patient is on a bed or chair from which he or she can rise only with great difficulty
- the patient feels weak and trembling; there is profuse sweating and a feverish feeling

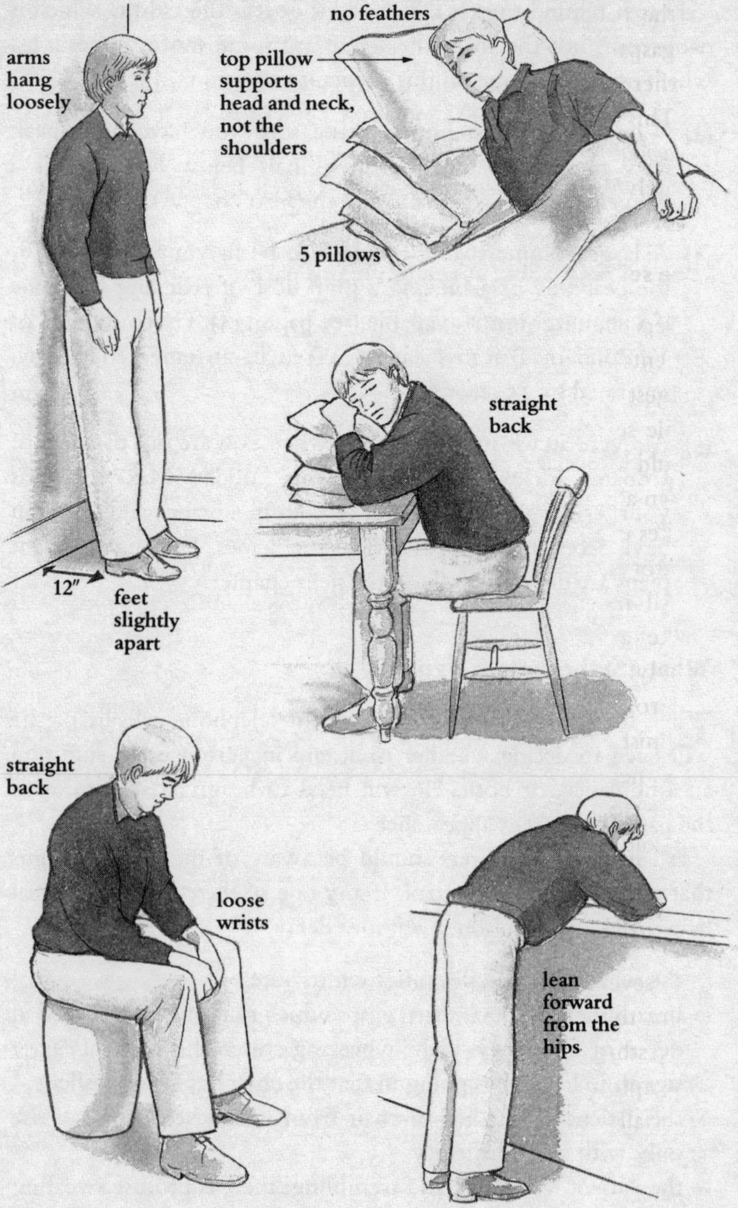

Fig. 16. Posture during an attack

- o the patient can utter only a few words, forced out between gasps
- o there is a blueness about the lips and tongue, or the fingernails. This is a signal of IMMEDIATE DANGER: *the next stage would be a sinking into unconsciousness*, so you should immediately dial 999 for an ambulance, as well as calling your doctor

The severe attack: some advice to carers

Carers should understand that, even in a severe attack, we patients want to make the least fuss possible. When the onlookers suggest sending for the doctor, we are likely to shake our heads while secretly hoping that this had already been arranged. We would also like a pencil and paper. If provided, we would write down a request for a glass of water (panting and profuse sweating makes us thirsty), and help so we can make an urgent visit to the lavatory, something we cannot manage on our own.

All medicines available should be at hand, to enable us to make a selection. We do *not* want advice about breathing slowly: the panting is probably automatic and beyond our control. We want help to be near, but not to be insistent or alarmist. When the ambulance arrives, it may help to take a dose of its nebulized salbutamol (or terbutaline) before being asked to make the difficult journey down the stairs and along the path in the cold, polluted air.

Posture during an attack

In a severe attack the patient tends to adopt the posture which seems to be most helpful. During a talk given to our branch of the Asthma Campaign, the Superintendent Physiotherapist at the Brompton Hospital in London explained that some postures, especially the sitting ones, are preferred when there is a severe attack:

1 Take the bronchodilator as prescribed.

2 Aim to breathe with minimum effort, so as to make the greatest use of the limited supply of oxygen.

3 Aim to relax the upper part of the chest and to relieve the pressure of the stomach on the diaphragm (this separates the lungs from the stomach). The method will depend on your situation. Five ways are shown in the illustration on page 141.

4 Breathe at your own rate. It may be easier to do this with the mouth open.

CHAPTER SEVEN

The Patient Takes Control

Patient, heal thyself?

In the past it has been common for doctors to ascribe poor control of asthma to 'non-compliance'. It seems that the fault lies not in our physicians but in ourselves that we continue to have troublesome symptoms!

Any reader of this book who has studied the previous chapters carefully may have concluded that compliance is desirable but only possible if certain conditions are fulfilled:

- the treatment has been fully explained, understood and accepted
- the way you use the inhaler has been checked
- the course of treatment has been written down in a comprehensible way
- the possible side-effects of the medicines have been described and are found to be acceptable
- enough medicine has been prescribed to last the course
- the treatment allows for adjustment by the patient to suit the day-to-day ups and downs of the illness
- the use of a peak flow meter has been explained, and the keeping of a daily record initiated

The invaluable peak flow meter

If your breathing tubes have become narrowed or partially

blocked, you will find it difficult to blow out hard. Your 'peak flow' will be diminished. A peak flow meter is a device which registers this expiratory peak flow on a scale. You blow into the mouthpiece as hard as you can; this pushes a needle along the scale, and the value is expressed in litres per minute. It is very easy to operate.

1 Stand up and hold the device level.
2 Take in a full breath – through the mouth or the nose – and gently fill out your chest until it will go no further (to 'total lung capacity').
3 While holding your breath, close your lips tightly around the mouthpiece, making sure that the meter's cursor is at the bottom.
4 Blow out as fast and as hard as you can through the mouthpiece and not at all through the nose. There is no need to empty your lungs.
5 On a meter designed for adults, the needle will stop somewhere between 60 and 800. On a meter made for children, the scale runs from 30 to 370.
6 Repeat the exercise twice, after a pause to recover your breath. Note all the readings and choose the *highest* (not the average) reading. This is usually the first of the readings.

Peak expiratory flow rate

You have just measured your **P.E.F.R.**, the shorthand for this section's title, in litres per minute. The peak flow meter is supplied with a chart which shows what people without asthma achieve, on average, according to sex, height and age. For example a male of my age and height should reach 560 litres a minute with a good strong blow. This is called my **predicted peak flow**: 560 litres of air would be blown out through the mouth in a minute.

As someone with severe and persistent asthma, my P.E.F.R.

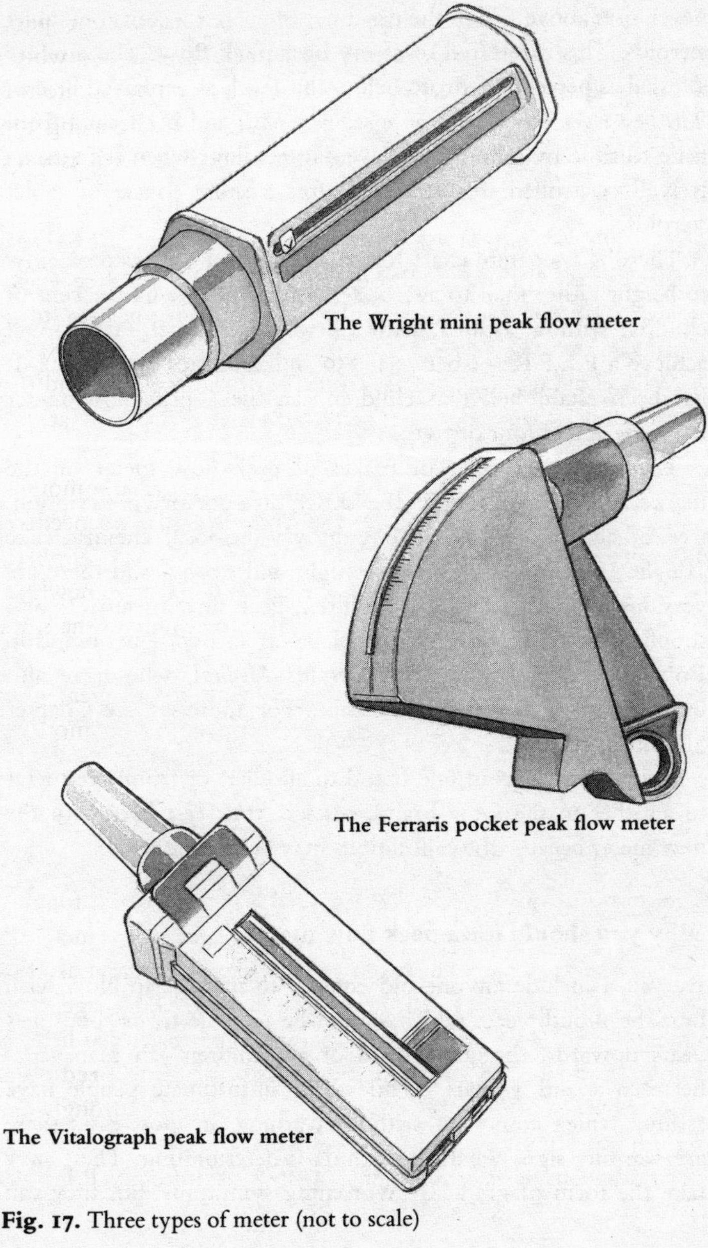

Fig. 17. Three types of meter (not to scale)

never rises above 350 in the daytime, even after a course of tablet steroids. This is referred to as my **best peak flow**. The dips are assessed as percentage drops below this level, as explained below. *The best level may change on a seasonal basis* and is checked from time to time by taking early evening readings when the asthma is well controlled, for example after a short course of tablet steroids.

There is a separate chart for children which relates peak flow to height rather than to age or sex – for example 95 per cent of children without asthma, with a height of 140 cm. (4′ 6″), will achieve a P.E.F.R. of between 250 and 400 litres per minute. It has been established that children can use a peak flow meter from the age of four or five.

There are a number of makes of peak flow meter on the market. All are available (in the U.K.), on a doctor's prescription, free of charge, or can be bought via the local chemist. The *Wright Mini Peak Flow Meter* is light and strong, and there are versions for both adults and children. Peak flow meters are also supplied by *Vitalograph* (also available as an own-label brand in Boots the Chemists) and by *Ferraris Medical*, who have also brought out a small pocket version. For addresses, see Chapter Seventeen.

If you change from one brand to another, or from one meter to another in the same brand, reassess your *best level* with the new meter because the calibrations may not be the same.

Why you should use a peak flow meter

By *you*, I include anyone old enough to manage to blow hard into the mouthpiece, which should be possible from about 4–5 years upwards, though a third of all children can manage at between 3 and 4 years. While some unfortunate people have asthma which comes on without warning, in most cases there are warning signs when the asthma is deteriorating. These may take the form of gradually worsening symptoms, but they can be misleading. By using a peak flow meter on a regular basis, you can confirm your subjective judgement:

- o if the gap between a.m. and p.m. readings is greater than 15 per cent . . .
- o if this gap is getting wider . . .
- o if either a.m. or p.m. (or both) readings are sliding downwards . . .

then you need either to seek medical help, or to change the treatment yourself according to a plan agreed in advance with your doctor.

There are other advantages of peak flow measurement. It can be used to pinpoint a trigger. A reading is taken when the suspected trigger is present and when it is absent, and the two results are compared. Peak flow readings can provide an objective assessment for parents of a child's asthma. They can help you plan the day, in so far as this is within your control, in conjunction with the weather forecast!

Deciding when to take readings

Some doctors ask patients to record peak flow three times a day. This is acceptable for a short period but if readings are to continue indefinitely, which is advisable for anyone who is taking *preventive* medicine on a regular basis, then morning and evening readings are adequate, taken before the *relieving* inhaler is used. You record the best of three readings, preferably with half a minute between them to allow for breathlessness caused by the reading itself.

Patients with mild asthma, with only a few occasional wheezes, need take readings only when the symptoms start to increase (for example during the summer pollen season).

The readings can be set down as numbers; for example:

	early morning	evening
day one	450	500
day two	425	480
day three	400	460
day four	375	440

In this example the readings are sliding downwards and the gap between morning and evening readings is increasing. The aim of treatment will be to reverse this slide and at the same time to move the early morning readings closer to those recorded before retiring to bed.

I find that my early morning readings climb steadily, even when a relieving medicine is not used, from (say) 250 at 6.30 a.m. to 310 at 8.30 a.m. So I try to fix on 8.00 a.m. in order to achieve consistency.

The diary card

Symptoms or peak flow readings noted at one moment only are not nearly as useful as those recorded over a period. This is why patients or parents are increasingly being asked to keep a daily record in the form of a diary, at least until the date fixed for the next medical consultation.

What is recorded will depend on the card that is used. The example given below is based on cards issued by two London hospitals. It enables the following information to be recorded, using numbers for the peak flow measurements, as in the example opposite:

- changes in symptoms
- activity
- peak flow meter readings
- the medicines used over the 24 hours
- comments such as (a) saw doctor; (b) absent from work/ school;

THE DIARY CARD

NAME .... **MONTH** .... **YEAR** ....

Date			1	2	3	4	5	6	7
last night	good night	0							
	slept well, slightly wheezy	1							
	woken 2–3 a.m.	2							
	bad: mostly awake	3							
wheeze last night	none	0							
	little	1							
	moderately bad	2							
	severe	3							
cough last night	none	0							
	occasional	1							
	frequent	2							
activity today	normal	0							
	can run a little	1							
	can only walk	2							
	off school or work	3							
peak flow	(best of 3 blows)								
	before a.m. medicine								
	before p.m. medicine								
medication	took as prescribed?								
	took extra doses?								
	took different med?								
	if so, which?								
additional info	runny nose?								
	itchy/puffy eyes?								
	weather change?								
	sore throat?								
	other illness?								
	saw the doctor?								
	travel away from home?								

Queries for the doctor

Fig. 18. Personal diary card

(c) any infection; (d) away from home; (e) any dramatic change in the weather (e.g. mist, thunder, a wet spell) that may have contributed

It takes only a few minutes to fill in the daily column, but the reward could be a marked improvement in treatment if the card is studied carefully by your doctor. It provides a common ground of information which all can share; it could also encourage the less confident to ask such questions as: 'You tell me that the medicine will enable me to lead a normal life but, doctor, is it really normal to wake up at 3 a.m. with a wheezy chest, two or three times a week?'

There is an added bonus! It is all too easy to forget to take the medicine that has been prescribed; this lapse has to be recorded on the card. Most asthmatics under-treat their asthma, and this may be corrected if a diary is kept. Make copies of the diary on page 149, try keeping the diary for a few weeks, and then show it to your general practitioner for his comments. If he tells you that you have been wasting your time, then you will at least have the private satisfaction of taking a contrary view!

Transferred to a chart

I find that the peak flow readings are much easier to interpret if they are transferred to a chart. Readings are plotted against peak flow numbers on the vertical axis and timings on the horizontal axis. These will show the best of morning and evening readings; afternoon measurements could be added as well. In the examples which follow, a continuous line is shown. An alternative would be to join the a.m. and the p.m. readings separately; this may be easier to interpret.

(1) The 'morning dipper' (Fig. 19)

Many asthmatics report that their worst symptoms are experienced when they wake up in the small hours of the morning.

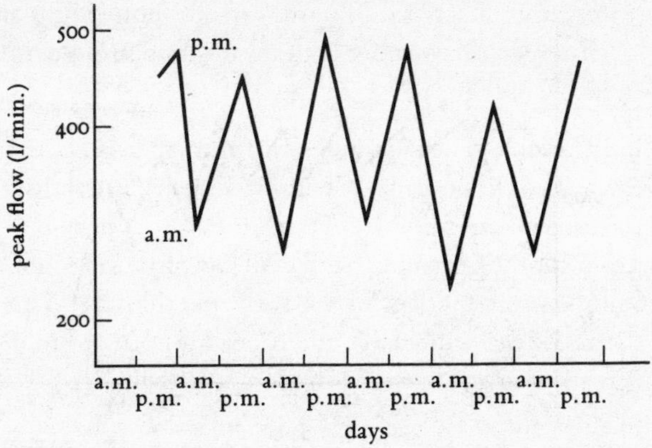

Fig. 19. Variations between a.m. and p.m. readings

This is known, not surprisingly, as 'the early morning dip'. The dip in peak flow will persist until the patient rises to begin the day's activities and takes the medicines. So night-time asthma is recorded as an 'a.m.' reading and daytime asthma as a 'p.m.' reading: confusing at first, but quite logical.

Figure 19 shows a regular fall in a.m. peak flow compared with the early evening reading which will register the daytime peak flow (asthma tends to improve during the day).

Even non-asthmatic people show a small reduction in peak flow at night and a drop of 15 per cent below the best daytime reading is acceptable. But in people with asthma which is poorly controlled, the gap can be as large as 50 per cent. It is an astonishing fact that lung function, as measured by peak flow, can drop significantly before some patients become aware that they have restricted breathing, especially when they are at rest. The aim of treatment will be to reduce the fall in peak flow so it is no greater than 15 per cent in the days which follow the treatment.

(2) The 'slow slider' (Fig. 20)

Patients get used to their symptoms and tolerate them, so they do not notice the slow deterioration until it is too late and they

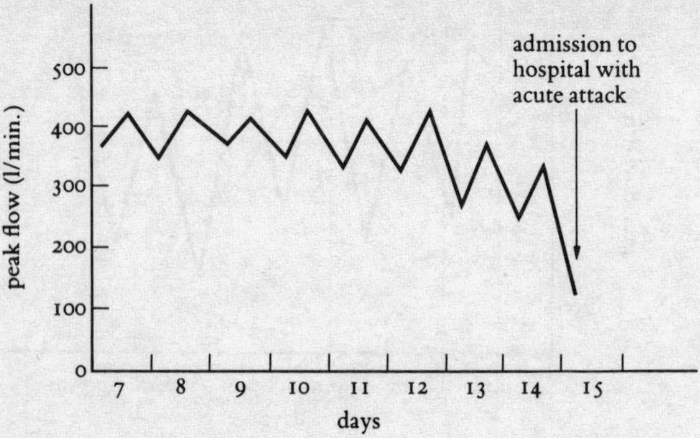

Fig. 20. Slow deterioration

find themselves in hospital after a most unnerving attack. If, on the other hand, we adopt the practice of keeping a diary of peak flow readings at times when we know we will be especially at risk (for example, in September when the children start again at school and spread infections around) then such a crisis can be anticipated, and we will change the treatment or consult the doctor in time to prevent the acute attack.

(3) Wheezy after exercise (Fig. 21)

When you turn up at the 5 p.m. surgery, you may show no sign of asthma. In order to confirm the diagnosis, the doctor may ask you to take vigorous exercise, having first taken a 'baseline' peak flow reading. The peak flow is recorded every minute after the exercise, for fifteen minutes, and a reliever is given to restore the normal function. The peak flow is measured; you run round the surgery for six minutes; then peak flow readings are taken.

Over 80 per cent of people with asthma will show a fall in peak flow of at least 15 per cent within ten minutes of stopping the exercise. The rapid improvement after a bronchodilator (reliever) has been used is another indicator that it is asthma.

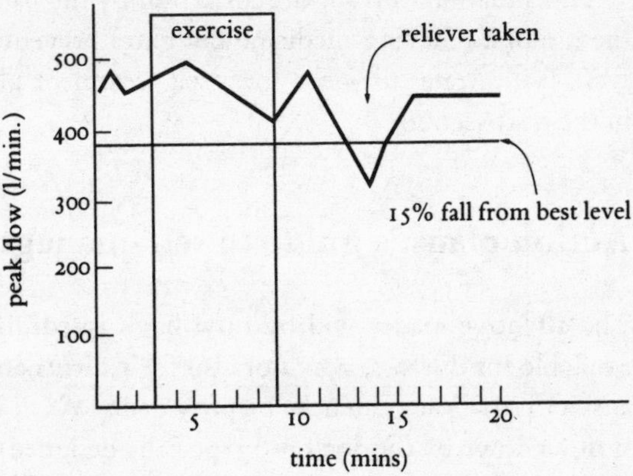

Fig. 21. Wheezy after exercise

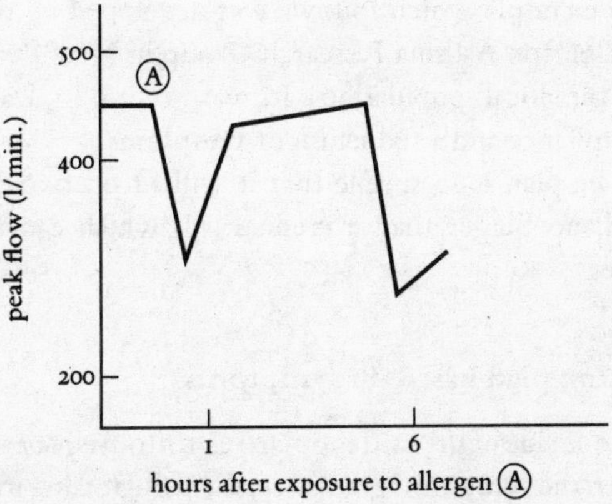

Fig. 22. A second-phase attack

(4) The second-phase attack (Fig. 22)

It is quite common for an attack of asthma to take place in two stages, as described in Chapter Two on page 29. The first attack subsides quite quickly and then, six hours later, is followed by asthma which is harder to control. This is because the swelling in the airways has increased. These stages will show up clearly from the peak flow readings, if taken at hourly intervals.

This situation calls for urgent action by the patient, not simply the use of a relieving medicine but extra preventive treatment as well. It illustrates the need for a self-treatment plan, as described in the next section.

Action plans: a guide to self-management

The attentive reader will by now have asked: 'If Guidelines are available for doctors, why not also for patients and parents?' The answer is that they can now be provided as ACTION PLANS, written down by the doctors on specially designed treatment cards.

These plans enable patients to adjust their treatment according to simple steps, based on the Guidelines described on page 129. The example which follows was developed by doctors from the Wellington Asthma Research Group in New Zealand, and tested on the local population. It was found to lead to improved compliance and a reduction of symptoms.

The plan is so simple that it will fit on two sides of a plastic card, no bigger than a credit card, which can be carried at all times.

Action plan based on symptoms

On one side of the card the plan relates to *symptoms*. The idea is that, when the symptoms get worse, the patient takes immediate action. In **step two** the dose of inhaled preventer will be doubled (this refers to inhaled steroid such as Becotide or Pulmicort). This is given a trial and, if unsuccessful, then **step three** is undertaken, a short course of tablet steroid (Prednisolone). At the same time the patient calls the doctor and in any case uses the reliever inhaler as needed.

Action plan based on peak flow readings

A better understanding of the state of the airways can be

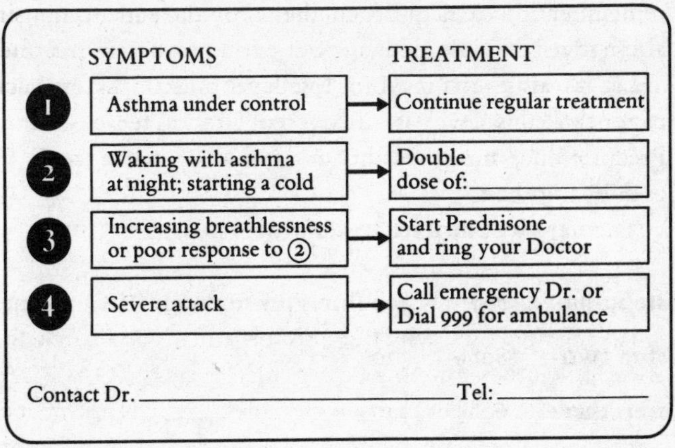

Fig. 23. Plastic treatment card

obtained if the steps are based on the a.m. and p.m. readings of peak flow measurement, as described on the previous pages. The steps are the same as in the example above (they are printed on the reverse of the card).

The best way to double the dose of inhaled steroid is to take a single puff every six hours. This may be hard for some of us to

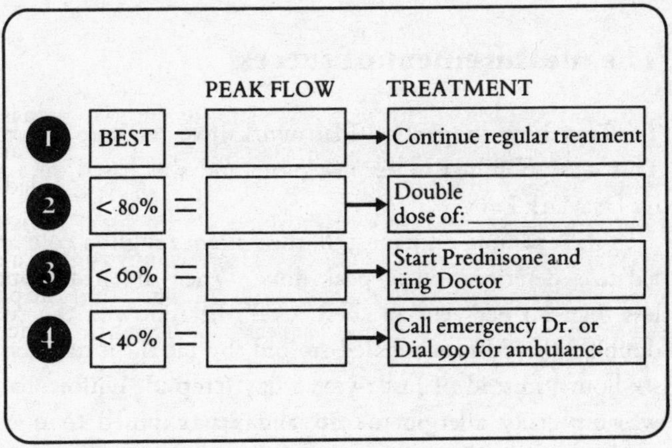

Fig. 24. Reverse of card

remember, so extra puffs in the morning and evening are an alternative.

Let us assume that your *best* level is 400. As explained on page 146, this level is discovered after a ten-day course on Prednisolone, measured in an afternoon, when peak flow is usually at its best.

The steps will then read as follows:

step one	*best*	400 (litres per minute)
step two	80%	320
step three	60%	240
step four	40%	160

These steps can be marked on a diary chart and projected forward so that you can see at a glance where the asthma is heading: they can be indicated in different colours.

The intervals of 80 per cent, 60 per cent and 40 per cent are arbitrary. Some patients may be better suited with different levels, as recommended by their physician.

The measurement of success

To show how the Action Plan works, we can take an example. This was published in *Asthma News* and was based on a lecture by Dr Mark Levy.

In the example on page 158, the patient caught a cold and this led to a deterioration in peak flow. When this had dropped to less than 80 per cent of 'best level', he followed the rule and doubled the dose of inhaled steroid, by taking it at intervals of six hours, instead of just twice a day (**step 2**). Unfortunately he was especially allergic to cats and was exposed to one when staying with a friend, so the peak flow level continued to drop.

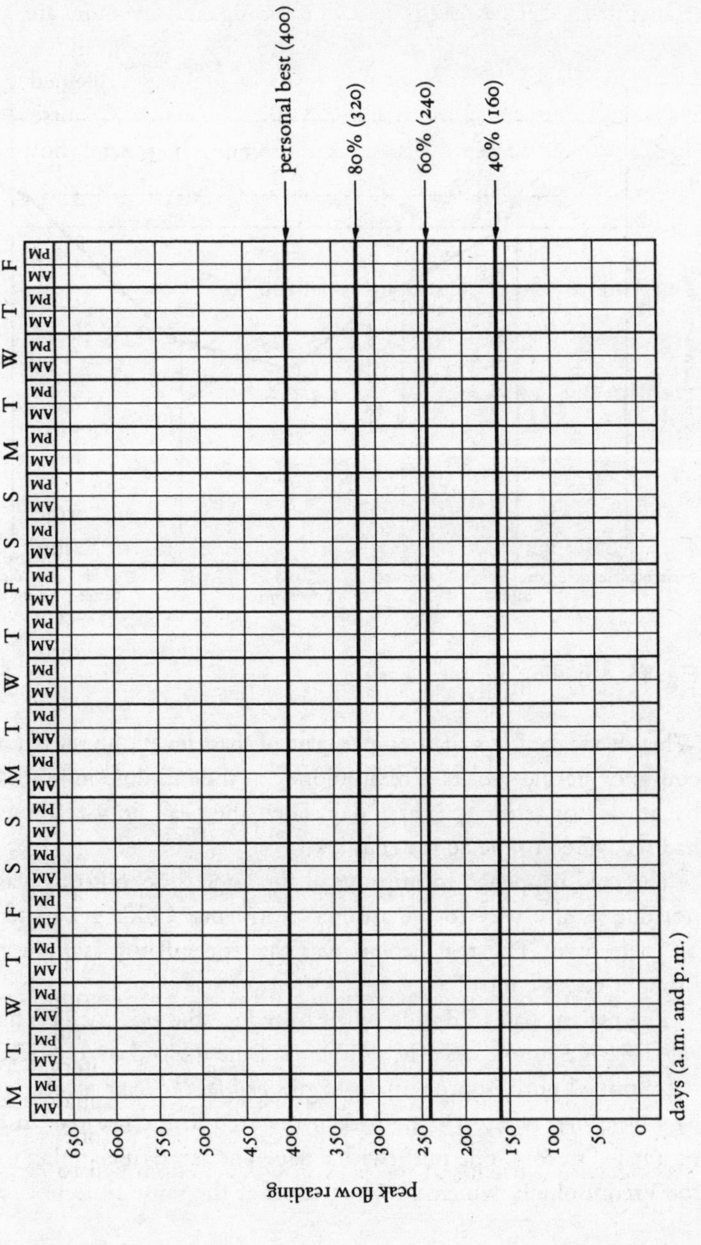

Fig. 25. Steps marked on a diary card, projecting forward, based on best = 400

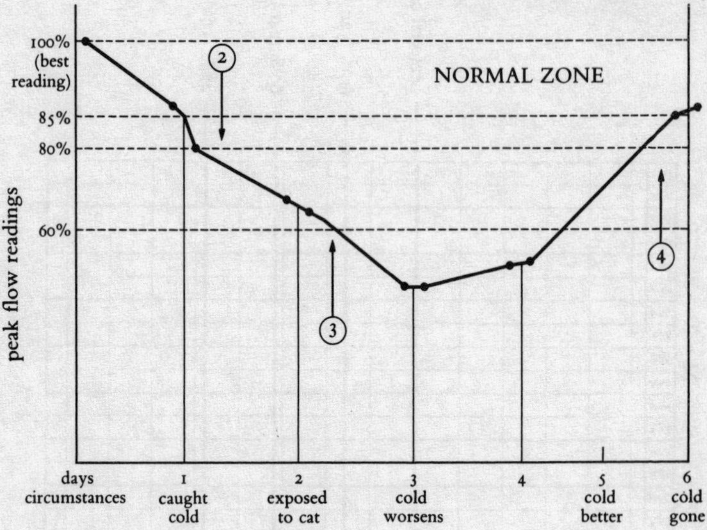

Fig. 26. Adjusting treatment in steps

When it reached less than 60 per cent of 'best level', he started a course of steroid tablets (Prednisolone), at the full dose indicated by his doctor (**step 3**). Three days later, the peak flow readings had recovered to the 80 per cent level.

The cold happened to improve at the same time, but this was not due in any way to the asthma treatments. Colds get better on their own. The real benefit was that the inflammation was brought under control.

The patient had to decide when to reduce the treatment. The rule here is a simple one: the doubling of the inhaled steroid dose is continued until improvement begins *and for the same number of days thereafter.* At **step 4** the patient reverted to the normal dose of inhaled steroid: one puff twice a day. The same rule applies to the Prednisolone, which is switched off at the same time but so as not to exceed a ten-day course. It is a good idea to keep it going for at least four days, as shown in the example, to make sure that the inflammation is well controlled.

The next **step** will be to consult your doctor, armed with the chart as a record, even if you have brought the attack under control. This is because a dangerously low level can be reached quite quickly, and there may be ways of avoiding a slide downwards in the future.

Asthma may change as time goes by, and your doctor may need to change the Action Plan, so a visit to the G.P. or nurse should be made at least twice a year.

Morning dippers and slow sliders

The self-management Action Plan can be applied to the charts on page 151–3. As far as 'morning dippers' are concerned, the aim will be to reduce the gap between a.m. and p.m. readings so that the drop between them is no greater than 15 per cent and, when this has been achieved, raise the p.m. readings so that they come close to the *best ever* level. One way of doing this may be to embark on a short (ten-day) course of tablet steroid (Prednisolone) and then to stabilize by twice-daily doses of inhaled steroid. If this does not help, then, as the Guidelines suggest on page 129, a slow-release reliever such as slow-release theophyline or salmeterol may be prescribed, and should be monitored on the diary card. I have noticed that this treatment has closed the gap between a.m. and p.m. readings but has not improved the level of p.m. results, evidence perhaps that inflammation has not been reduced.

Deterioration in peak flow readings may be very gradual, as illustrated on page 152 (Fig. 20). You have become a 'slow slider'. No moral blame attaches, unless you fail to take the remedy indicated on the Action Plan: to increase the dose of inhaled steroid when the reading reaches the 80 per cent level and add Prednisolone if the 60 per cent level is being indicated by your peak flow readings.

Combining diary and chart

If you decide to discuss the chart with your doctor, then a record of the medicine taken will help him to adjust the treatment plan, if need be.

All you have to record is the number of puffs each day of (a) *preventer* inhaler, and (b) *reliever* inhaler, plus (c) the number of Prednisolone tablets if that **step** has been reached. These can be entered at the foot of the chart each day and will help you to remember to take the treatments.

An additional piece of information could be a note (in code) of any major changes in the *triggers*: 'Inf' = caught a cold; 'CA' = cold air; 'Pol' = high pollen count; 'Cat' = met a cat.

It is surprising how quickly these details can be entered and how much you can learn about ways of bringing the asthma under control. The chart soon fills up, so make a few copies from the empty master when next at the copy shop. The chart should be kept going in good times and in bad, otherwise how will you be able to detect the slow slide or the increasing 'morning dip'? But do not emulate the lady who waited five years before submitting 87 charts to her physician!

Do not rely on the charts alone. If symptoms have deteriorated, do not wait until 60 per cent has been reached on the chart before switching to the emergency plan. It is a good idea to record symptoms as well, in code, on the sheet. For example: 'SL' = loss of sleep; 'BE' = breathless through exercise.

Conclusion

It takes only a few minutes to take a reading and record it on a chart. The benefits greatly outweigh this small effort. You become more aware of the way the triggers act on the airways, better able to predict their response, and much more likely to be able to modify this response through an enlightened choice of treatment. It also helps you remember to take the treatments!

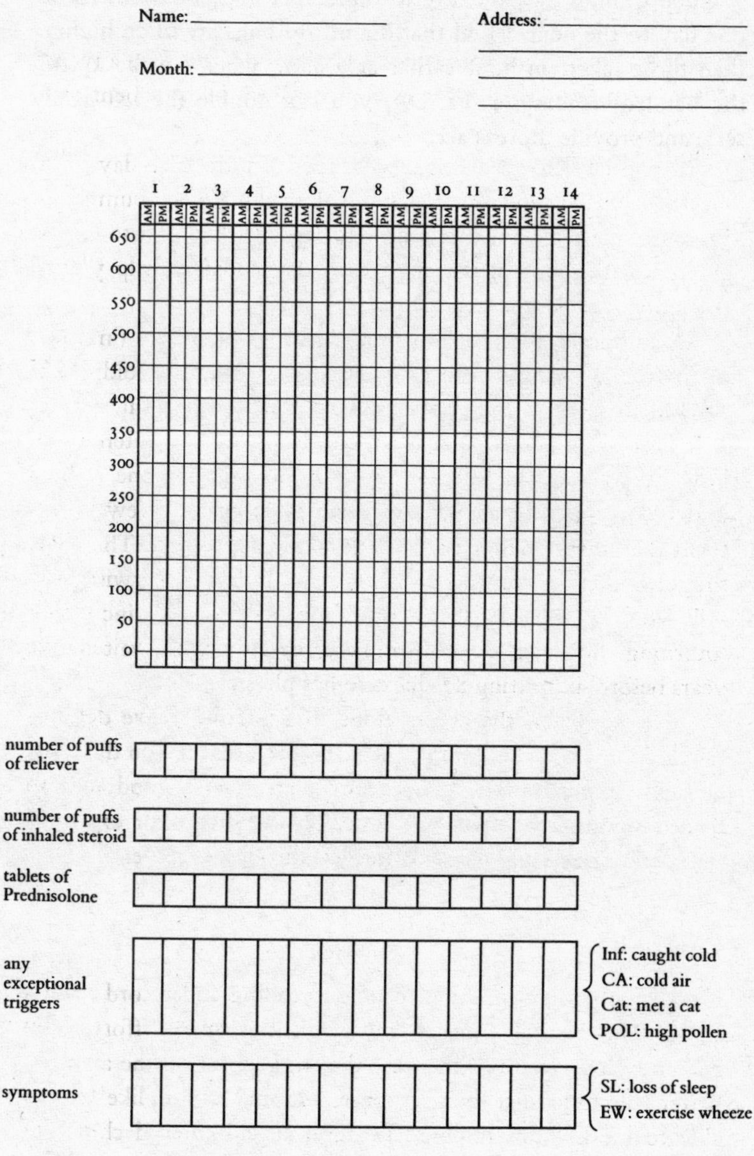
Name:
Address:
Month:
1 2 3 4 5 6 7 8 9 10 11 12 13 14
AM PM
650
600
550
500
450
400
350
300
250
200
150
100
50
0
number of puffs of reliever
number of puffs of inhaled steroid
tablets of Prednisolone
any exceptional triggers
Inf: caught cold
CA: cold air
Cat: met a cat
POL: high pollen
symptoms
SL: loss of sleep
EW: exercise wheeze

Fig. 27. Combined chart and diary

Choose times that are easy to remember and consistent from one day to the next. I find that 8 a.m. readings are often higher than those taken an hour earlier at 7 a.m., when I wake up. If the band of readings is narrow, you can double the left-hand scale and provide more space.

CHAPTER EIGHT

Living with an Asthmatic Child

A series of challenges

The parents' first reaction to a diagnosis that their child has asthma is likely to be one of shock and uncertainty. What does the future hold in store? Is the child going to suffer a lifetime of illness? In reality, if the asthma is typical of that of the majority, it will be mild, occasional and manageable with simple treatments, which will allow the child to lead a full and normal life. Even so, the parents will still have to adjust to those sudden and alarming attacks of breathlessness, to the paroxysms of night coughing and to the child's silent appeals for help when there seems to be no immediate improvement.

Living with asthma in the family presents many challenges. Not the least of these is that it is hard to judge the seriousness of the attack and to know when you need to summon a doctor. There are worries about the medicines, and there may be difficulty in persuading the child to take them. There are countless anxieties as to what may be causing the asthma and, perhaps associated with this, a feeling of guilt that not enough is being done to remove the causes.

The parents are not likely to receive much help from family and friends if these people have not had experience of the illness. Asthma tends either to be dismissed as a trivial complaint, easily reversed with modern medicines, or to be seen as a nervous condition, made worse by 'over-protection'. The parents are advised by those around them to wait until the child grows out of the asthma, and in the meantime simply to put up with it.

The family doctor will be able to set the record straight and provide that badly needed reassurance. But doctors are under pressure; consultations can be hurried affairs and often leave the parents as confused as ever, so that they sometimes feel isolated and threatened. Friendships are put to the test and the marriage itself may come under strain through the stress of coping with the illness.

A common illness

It may be of some comfort to be reminded that asthma is one of the most common illnesses in childhood. It affects one child in ten and is responsible, more than any other illness, for keeping children away from school. It is not therefore surprising that self-help groups have been formed which enable parents to share their experiences with one another. At the time of writing, the National Asthma Campaign in the U.K. has nearly 200 branches, and there are similar voluntary organizations in many other countries (see Chapter Fourteen and Chapter Seventeen, Useful Addresses).

Children themselves, with their enormous vitality, are pretty resilient. They come to accept asthma as the normal way of life, the only one known to them. The attacks may be terrifying, their outcome seemingly uncertain – but they are soon forgotten when breathing becomes normal again. Children learn to accept the constraints that asthma imposes, and adapting to it presents a challenge, along with all the other challenges they meet as they grow up.

How can the doctor tell it is asthma?

Parents may become alarmed when told that their child has asthma. This has led some doctors to use instead rather meaningless phrases such as 'wheezy bronchitis' or 'wheezy chest'. This concealment of the truth may have the unfortunate result that the parents will suspect that something is being hidden from them, that the illness is more severe than is really the case. It can also lead to inappropriate treatments. In a study, now famous in medical circles, which was carried out in Newcastle-upon-Tyne in 1983, all the children aged seven were examined in a large area of the city. It was found that out of 176 children who were wheezy, only 21 had been told that they had asthma. Once they had been started on the proper asthma treatment, the amount of schooling lost greatly decreased.

1 Does the wheeziness or tightness get worse at night, often just before going to sleep and just before waking up?

2 Does the wheeziness or tightness become worse following exercise? If the answer is a definite 'yes', then this is a certain sign of asthma. If there is no clear answer, the child may be asked by the doctor to run up and down the street, or to use an exercise bicycle, with readings of peak flow taken before and after to see if this has diminished as a result of the exercise.

3 Does the wheeziness or tightness disappear within a few minutes of taking a couple of puffs from a relieving inhaler (bronchodilator)?

4 Do attacks tend to follow a virus infection such as a head cold?

5 Has the child missed odd days from school because of chest symptoms?

If the answer to any of these questions is 'yes', then the child *probably* has asthma.

The questions that parents often ask

I have already dealt with questions concerning asthma and heredity in Chapter Two. A tendency to have an atopic illness (i.e. due to allergy) such as asthma, eczema, hay fever, urticaria (nettle rash) or migraine tends to run in families. The chance that a child will develop an atopic illness of one kind or another is about 12 per cent if neither parent has 'atopy', 25 per cent if one parent has atopic symptoms, and 50 per cent if these have appeared in both parents. About 40 per cent of asthmatic children also develop eczema, an illness which is beyond the scope of this book but which is covered in the list of Useful Addresses in Chapter Seventeen. This leads to our first question.

Should we have children?

The fact that there is a relative on both sides of the family with severe asthma does not mean that the children will have asthma which is severe. It is more likely to be mild and therefore easy to manage. If one child already has asthma, there can be no guarantee that the next will be free – but the chances are in favour of this being so.

How can we protect babies from triggers?

In order to reduce as far as possible the load of challenges which the new-born child has to face, an ultra-sensible couple might decide to avoid times of birth which will coincide with the peak pollen season (June and July) or the peak mould season (the summer holidays) or the peak time for house dust mites (autumn and early winter). This would leave 'clear' January to March. However, there is as yet no evidence that babies born at this time are less prone to allergic illnesses. It is the *first six months* of the infant's life that are critical.

If a mother comes from a family with a history of allergy, or if she has been told that she has a higher-than-average level of

IgE antibody in the blood and a lower-than-average level of the 'T-cells' which suppress these antibodies, what can she do? As explained below, breast feeding may help. In the critical first six months, allergens and irritants should be avoided wherever possible: no animals; total war on airborne allergens, especially the house dust mite, and the ban on cigarettes continued. Some allergists would also add advice about diet.

Does asthma cause problems in pregnancy?

Many pregnant women find that their asthma improves during pregnancy, and others do not notice any change. It is unusual for asthma to worsen during pregnancy. Any improvement will be due to an increase in the production of steroid by the mother's adrenal glands.

The health of a new-born baby is unlikely to be affected by the mother's asthma, and the risk of a severe attack during labour itself is extremely low because the adrenal glands pour out cortisone and adrenaline into the blood. To reduce the risk of a severe attack, the preventer medicines should be taken, as prescribed.

Can the drugs used in asthma affect pregnancy?

The adrenaline derivatives, such as salbutamol and terbutaline, are sometimes used by obstetricians to try to prevent premature labour, but in very high doses; when used to treat asthma in much lower doses, they do not have this effect. Theophylline (but not aminophylline) has been found to be safe in pregnancy. Intal appears to be safe in every condition. This leaves the steroids. They should preferably be taken only in inhaled doses. Tablet steroids can be used in pregnancy, though the drug could reach the baby in small amounts.

Remember to include the inhalers in your maternity packing.

Is breast feeding desirable?

There is strong evidence that breast feeding, continued for six months, will reduce the chance of a baby later becoming allergic to cow's milk and developing eczema. Since eczema is a possibility when either parent is 'atopic' (has an allergy), breast feeding is preferable. It may delay but is unlikely to prevent the onset of asthma (see page 213).

While breast feeding, you can continue to take both relievers and preventers, from inhalers. If you use a spacer canister (see page 115), then the chance of any drug being swallowed and absorbed into the circulation and appearing in the breast milk will be extremely small.

Do children change their sensitivities?

The commonest cause of wheezing that lasts for more than a few days is a viral infection of the nose (and often of the throat as well), especially in the first three years of life. This occurs most often in families with no history of asthma, is not allergic and is mostly outgrown by school age. It seems that not only are antibiotics useless; there are no adequate vaccines either – and in any case the child must develop his or her own immunity.

In young children asthma is more often revealed through coughing than through wheezing, always worse at night. Exercise usually makes the asthma worse, and in half the children excitement and emotional upsets are triggers.

In older children, of school age, allergy plays an important part. Half of *all* children would show up as positive on a skin prick test to at least one allergen, even though only 10 per cent of children develop asthma; many others are what doctors describe as 'nosey'.

Food intolerance rarely plays a part in older children. The main trigger, until puberty, is the house dust mite. Then, as a result of continuous exposure to it, children come to tolerate it to some extent. Then the various pollens and moulds tend to take over as the most common allergic triggers. It is more difficult to acquire a tolerance of these because they come and go on a seasonal basis.

Can asthma affect growth?

It is usually the case in children with atopy (an allergic illness), especially if it is persistent, that in the early teens their increase in height seems to be less than that of their friends, due to a slight delay in the onset of puberty. However, they all catch up when the growth spurt is completed, so why worry? The children worry because for a time they seem to be small by comparison, can no longer compete in sports and their self-confidence and concentration at school work may diminish.

The cause of this delay is not known. It takes place in all children with atopy, whether or not they have asthma, and has nothing to do with the severity, the diet or the medicines that are taken.

Normal people release lots of growth hormone during the earlier part of the night during sleep and little thereafter. But children with asthma release hormones in small spurts throughout the night, and also under the stress of asthma. The result is that they may well end up taller than their friends who do not have asthma, provided they have a healthy balanced diet and a good control over their asthma.

Can medicines affect growth?

Studies have shown that inhaled steroids, up to a maximum dosage of 800 micrograms of Becotide a day, have no effect on growth, even when they are taken throughout childhood. This is because they have a low 'bio-availability'. This means that, if swallowed, very little of the drug reaches the general circulation. This is especially true of Flixotide and Pulmicort, the inhaled steroids with the lowest bio-availability, for a given dose.

In higher doses there *could* be an influence on the way bone is set down, so it is essential that the drug be delivered as efficiently as possible into the airways, especially as children vary greatly in their tolerance of the steroids.

Will my child grow out of asthma?

Far fewer adults have asthma than children. If the asthma is due to wheezy viral infections in infancy, there is a good chance that it will disappear at around five years of age.

Atopic (allergic) asthma in schoolchildren often improves at puberty, or in the late teens. If the asthma is severe and persistent in childhood, there is a greater likelihood that it will reappear at some time in later life. However, the use of modern preventive medicines may improve the outlook, and parents should make sure that they are taken regularly and properly.

Why should smoking be avoided?

If the mother smokes during pregnancy, the harmful chemicals can be absorbed by the unborn child. There is growing evidence that smoking in pregnancy interferes with the child's lung development and can lead to asthma in infancy when there are virus infections, or to other allergies developing later in childhood. A low weight at birth can be caused by the mother's smoking, and in turn can contribute to asthma later on. The child, at any age, should be protected from passive inhalation of other people's cigarette smoke. After infancy smoke can be a trigger. Children copy their parents. By the age of sixteen a quarter of all children in the United Kingdom are regular smokers.

Is vaccination safe?

Whooping cough, with its prolonged fits of racking cough, is particularly dangerous for a child with asthma. They can cause a child to vomit and, in extreme circumstances, to stop breathing. Even when an attack is in progress, children with asthma can be vaccinated against whooping cough, and for all the other routine immunizations, plus those carried out before travelling abroad. This is also the case with other forms of allergy (hay fever, eczema, etc.). Modern vaccines are no longer dangerous in the child who is sensitive to eggs. The 'MMR' vaccine (measles, mumps and rubella) may not be suitable if the child is sick with a fever or on a course of steroid tablets; for these and similar precautions, consult your doctor.

Are boys and girls equally likely to develop asthma?

It is a remarkable and so far unexplained fact that, in childhood asthma, boys outnumber girls by two to one up to the age of thirteen years. After that, the girls catch up with the boys. In the more severe forms, boys predominate. It is not known why this should be so.

Hormonal factors affecting asthma can also be seen in the menstrual cycle, especially if the asthma is severe. It may get worse in the week before a period, and then improve during the early part of the cycle. It can be treated with progesterone. Self-management would be helped by increasing preventer medicine when a fall in peak flow is expected.

Is chest deformity common?

This used to be a common feature of children with severe and persistent asthma. Nowadays this is rare because this kind of asthma can be controlled with inhaled steroids. The existence of chest deformity can be taken as a sign of incorrect treatment. Fortunately it can be reversed after a year or two.

Do some medicines make children excitable?

Relievers (Ventolin and Bricanyl) taken as a syrup may cause a tremor in the hands and a racing of the heart. In a few instances it can make a child hyperactive. Inhaled relievers are unlikely to cause these problems, except at high doses, which are not normally needed. The use of spacers is described in Chapter Five.

Can I give my child an overdose?

The relievers (Ventolin and Bricanyl) administer very small inhaled doses and you have to take 15 and 30 puffs respectively before you reach a single dose from a nebulizer. The prescribed dose of theophyllines (e.g. Nuelin, Slo-Phylline, etc.) should never be exceeded, and blood tests are advisable from time to time to ensure that the blood levels are not too high. They are not used in young children.

Excessive use of relievers means that the asthma is poorly controlled: talk to your doctor about adding (or changing or increasing) *preventive* medicine. Intal and Tilade are entirely safe at any dose level. As far as inhaled steroids are concerned, their effectiveness is not increased beyond the maximum recommended dose. Tablet steroids are designed for short courses.

Should we consider a special school?
It is possible to send your child to a special school, such as the Pilgrim's School near Brighton, which takes children with severe and persistent asthma. No fees are paid by parents (local authorities are asked to contribute). Far from being over-protected at the school, the children manage through expert care to cast aside what may have been a crippling disability and learn to excel in all the activities that healthy children enjoy. Children with severe asthma who are very unhappy at their present school or who are unable to cope at home benefit greatly from being able to mix and compete with other children on equal terms.

The questions children ask

I enjoy giving talks to children in schools. One of the questions they ask is whether asthma is 'catching'. It is not. However, respiratory infections are passed around the school and these can lead to wheeziness. The question I used to ask *myself* in childhood was 'why me?' It is essential to remove any feeling of guilt and to emphasize that asthma is due to extra sensitivity to those mysterious airborne triggers.

The principles of management

Managing asthma in infants

When a baby enters the world following its sheltered life in the womb, it has to adapt to a place where many decisions have to be made. It has to distinguish between things which are good for it (such as food) and things which are bad for it (such as germs and toxic substances). It develops an immune system whereby injurious particles are attacked, surrounded and overwhelmed, while harmless and beneficial substances are accepted and tolerated. Some babies decide that particles entering their airways are harmful and thus become wheezy or develop a night cough, even though the particles could easily be cleared through the wafting of mucus up and out of the airways.

The most common form of wheezing in young children, particularly in the first year or two of life, is that they have one or two attacks which follow virus infections, like a cold. Instead of just having stuffed-up noses, some babies have a similar problem in their chests. Their airways are tiny anyway, so this can lead to coughs, wheezes or shortness of breath.

Other triggers can include exercise, excitement and even crying. Smoking by the mother before birth or in the home by anybody, the presence of pets, and damp housing can lead to asthma in infancy.

Persistent asthma in infants is rare. If symptoms are severe then a visit to a hospital is indicated, especially as asthma in infants is often missed or treated inappropriately. Time is the best healer and about 80 per cent of infants grow out of their asthma by the time they are five years old.

Giving medicine to infants

The medicines used are similar to those used in adult asthma. Atrovent is often prescribed as a reliever, effective in about 40 per cent of infants. The most appropriate way of delivering the medicines, whether relievers or preventers, is by using a spacer with a face-mask attached (see Fig. 28). The canister is held in a tilted position so that the valve stays open. If this is not available, then an inhaler inserted into the base of a large paper or plastic coffee cup and placed over the baby's face is a practical alternative. A

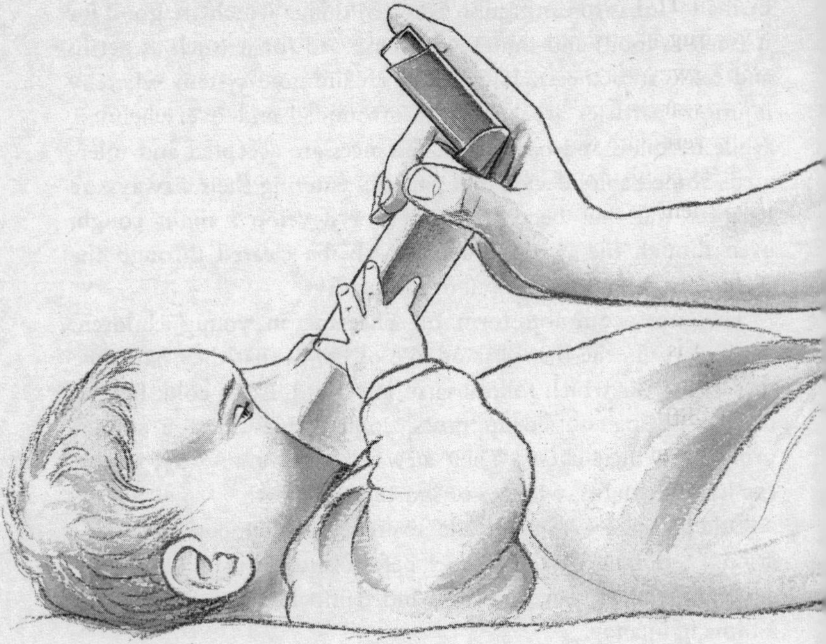

Fig. 28. The Aerochamber spacer (Medic-Aid)

large-volume spacer with the mouthpiece removed can also be used. If the spacer is suitably decorated it can become a toy (a spaceship when used by older children!). The medicine can be given even when the child is crying.

Over the age of three most children can use a mouthpiece. Nebulizers are rarely needed, and tablets are given only when the asthma is mild. As children develop, they can manage an increasing variety of inhaler treatments. Some mothers worry that inhalers are too powerful for young children. They can be reassured: inhalers are designed to *reduce* the amount of drug which is given, well below that which is needed in syrups or tablets.

Some mothers find it easier to give medicines in the form of a syrup. This has the disadvantage that, in common with tablets, the drug has to circulate round the bloodstream before it reaches the airways. It is a slow process and, when used in this way, side-effects are more likely. So doctors try to persuade parents to persevere with the inhalers.

The cough mixtures available at present have no place in the treatment of asthma, as explained on page 107.

Two related illnesses

Croup is also caused by common colds and takes the form of a barking cough and 'crowing' noise in young children. It may cause difficulty in breathing but does not usually lead to asthma. Asthma must not be confused with bronchiolitis, a viral chest infection which can affect infants under six months old and which results in wheeze and cough which persist for many months.

Avoiding the triggers

Although asthma in infancy is usually caused by infections, recent research has tended to confirm that the first year of life is the one in which the child is most likely to become sensitized to allergens, even though allergic asthma does not appear until later, perhaps many years later.

A trial arranged by Dr David Hide on the Isle of Wight, England, aimed to reduce both dietary and air-borne triggers in a group of new-born babies who were considered, from their family history, to be at a high risk of developing asthma, eczema and other diseases associated with allergy.

Dr Hide explained: 'The diet of lactating mothers was adjusted to avoid all milk and milk products, fish, eggs and nuts up to nine months or until lactating ceased, with supplementary calcium and vitamins. Alternatively, the infants were fed with a "low-allergenic" formula. Foods which are potentially allergenic were introduced in stages into the child's diet after nine months.

'At the same time efforts were made to reduce exposure to house dust mite by nursing the children on covered mattresses and by treating the bedroom and living-room carpets and the upholstered furniture with an anti-mite preparation.

'Children in this intervention group showed substantially less asthma, eczema or other allergy than a control group in the two years after birth. They appeared significantly less sensitized to both foods and airborne allergens. The trial continues.'

The triggers are described in detail in Chapter Three. One which applies to infants only is that the move away from high prams to low open buggies increases a child's exposure to vehicle exhaust fumes at ground level.

Managing asthma after infancy

The principles are the same as when managing asthma in adults: parents must start a dialogue with the doctor or nurse which will enable the treatments to be used effectively, with a 'crisis' plan worked out in advance should the asthma suddenly get worse. The special problems that arise with children relate to their inability to report on their illness and to take the medicines on their own initiative.

We have already studied the possible ways of reducing the triggers. The points that need emphasizing where children are concerned are that the bedroom should be kept as free as possible from house dust and animals, that smoking should be banned and that, when parties and special occasions are being planned, the preparations should be kept in a low key, since attacks can be brought on by excitement.

What are the warning signs? It is always easier to deal with an attack in the early stages, and any of the following signs may be taken as an indication, in a child prone to asthma, that an attack is under way:

- a persistent cough
- a runny, then a stuffed-up nose (i.e. starting a cold)
- irritability
- a disinclination to eat
- breathlessness following any increase in physical activity such as climbing the stairs
- a tendency to become easily tired and lethargic
- wheeziness
- some difficulty in talking
- itching, known as 'prodromal itching', can occur before an attack, usually in the same part of the body each time. The child is unlikely to mention it without prompting

In the classroom the teacher may detect a lack of concentration, and the child may sit at the desk with hunched shoulders.

Asthma treatment cards

It is usually difficult to remember any treatment plan which has not been fully explained and written down. The National Asthma Campaign can provide a card on which the plan can be set down. This will note day-to-day treatment and also suggest a 'crisis plan'. It is essential that it should be reviewed with the doctor or nurse every few months (see pages 178-9).

Using a peak flow meter

Anyone who has read the previous chapters will be in no doubt that regular checks with a peak flow meter can help improve both the understanding and the management in many ways. If readings are taken when the child is well, this will provide a benchmark or 'best level' against which to judge future readings. There is a special Mini-Wright peak flow meter which is designed for children. At what age can they begin to use one? They start to be useful from four or five years onwards. Some

WHAT TO DO FOR AN ATTACK

1. Relief treatment can be used
   - before known triggers, such as exercise, parties, smoky places
   - to relieve sudden wheeze and cough, such as after exercise or in the night
   - to relieve attacks lasting for a day or more, such as during a cold or at certain seasons
2. Repeat relief treatment if necessary (or if peak flow is in mild to moderate range
3. If no improvement or worsening after 2 doses of reliever, then
   - start steroid (Prednisolone) therapy as instructed
   - or ....
4. If symptoms remain severe (peak flow in severe range)
   - call your GP or go to the nearest Hospital Accident and Emergency Department or dial 999 for an ambulance
   - repeat your reliever (or nebulizer) while waiting
   - start steroid (Prednisolone) therapy or follow other instructions provided: ....

....

5

CARD CHECKED:

Date	Initials	Date	Initials

Take this card with you when you go to see *any* doctor or Asthma Clinic. It must be filled in or altered when treatment is changed.

NATIONAL **ASTHMA** CAMPAIGN
getting your breath back

Providence House, Providence Place, London N1 0NT.
Tel: 071–226 2260.
Asthma Helpline: 0345–01 01 03 (1 p.m. to 9 p.m., Mon. – Fri.).

6

CHILD'S ASTHMA CARD

Name ______________________
Address ______________________
____
____
Tel. No.:
Home ______________________
Parents' work ______________________
General Practitioner ______________________
Address ______________________
____
Tel. No. ______________________
Consultant ______________________
Hospital ______________________
Hospital Reference No. ______________________
Tel. No. ______________________

Always keep this card handy. Take it with you everywhere you go

1

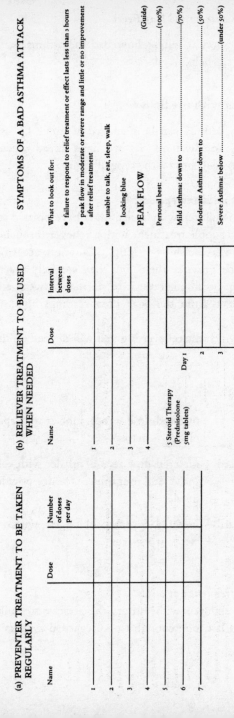

(a) PREVENTER TREATMENT TO BE TAKEN REGULARLY

	Name	Dose	Number of doses per day
1			
2			
3			
4			
5			
6			
7			

2

(b) RELIEVER TREATMENT TO BE USED WHEN NEEDED

	Name	Dose	Interval between doses
1			
2			
3			
4			

5 Steroid Therapy (Prednisolone 5mg tablets)

Day 1		
2		
3		
4		

3

SYMPTOMS OF A BAD ASTHMA ATTACK

What to look out for:

- failure to respond to relief treatment or effect lasts less than 3 hours
- peak flow in moderate or severe range and little or no improvement after relief treatment
- unable to talk, eat, sleep, walk
- looking blue

PEAK FLOW (Guide)

Personal best: ....(100%)

Mild Asthma: down to ....(70%)

Moderate Asthma: down to .... (50%)

Severe Asthma: below ....(under 50%)

Fig. 29. Treatment card devised by the National Asthma Campaign for doctors to set out the treatment plan. An adult card is also available

families are not good at telling how bad the asthma is, and a peak flow meter can help.

Treating asthma with medicines

In most children, asthma can be managed at home by using a variety of simple medications. As we have already seen, the choice of medicine depends on the type of asthma.

Asthma which is mild and episodic

Three-quarters of children who have asthma have isolated attacks which respond to simple treatment with a reliever (bronchodilator). The attacks may be short or long in duration, according to the triggers which provoke them, but they are fully reversible: that is to say, the breathing returns to normal between attacks. This can be judged from the peak flow readings in the older children.

The form in which the reliever is given will depend on the age of the child:

approximate age	
infancy	metered-dose aerosol inhaler with spacer, plus face-mask
3 years and upwards	metered-dose aerosol inhaler with valved spacer and mouthpiece, or dry powder inhaler
5 years and upwards	metered-dose aerosol inhaler, with or without a spacer

The attacks are frequent but mild

In a quarter of children with asthma the attacks are mild but frequent and can last long enough to be regarded as 'persistent', especially if peak flow readings do not return to normal in between attacks. (In the four case studies in Chapter Six, Mary provides an example of this kind of asthma.)

The persistence calls for regular preventive treatment. The medicine tried first is sodium cromoglycate (Intal or Cromolyn), which is effective in a majority of children with persistent asthma. If this proves to be ineffective, an inhaled steroid (e.g. Becotide, Flixotide or Pulmicort) is used from a large-volume spacer, on a regular basis. In addition, the inhaled reliever (Ventolin, Bricanyl or Aerolin) is taken as needed, and also before play or exercise. The asthma is checked from time to time with a peak flow meter. If the peak flow returns to normal and stays there for a few months, then the preventive treatment may be discontinued, on a trial basis.

The attacks are infrequent but severe

Some asthmatic children have attacks which occur less frequently than, say, once a month, but they are sometimes severe. Between the attacks the children are free from wheeze and breathlessness, and peak flow readings return to normal. In these cases the inhaled bronchodilator may not be capable of reversing the attacks, even at twice the normal dose. Possible treatments include the use of a nebulizer to provide a much higher dose of bronchodilator, or a short course of steroid in tablet form, in order to restore peak flow to normal. The steroid course will run for only 3–4 days, and no permanent side-effects will be experienced. If neither of these treatments is available, then the doctor should be consulted.

The attacks are both persistent and severe

In a very small proportion of asthmatic children, perhaps under 5 per cent of all children with asthma, the attacks are frequent, prolonged and often severe, and the peak flow readings never reach what is normal for the age of the child. In such cases the very high responsiveness has to be damped down with anti-inflammatory medicine, taken night and morning in the form of an inhaled steroid (an example of this condition has already been given in the case studies, that of Anthony).

Activities have to be restricted to those which can be tolerated. There are likely to be some admissions to hospital; in between the worst episodes, a regular check at the surgery or clinic will be essential, to ensure that the best possible treatment is being given at home and is being taken in the correct way. A crisis plan, with the appropriate medicine, is essential.

The aim in treatment will be to rescue the child as rapidly as possible from the severe attack, using either steroid tablets in high dosage or a nebulized bronchodilator or both. The second aim will be to lift the whole day and night peak flow pattern to a new and higher level, by the use of the inhaled steroid, initially at a high dose and then reduced until a maintenance level is reached, so that the pattern is closer to the normal.

In spite of their disability, even children in this severe category do manage to lead fairly normal lives and take part in outdoor activities which are moderately strenuous, so building up their physical, mental and moral strength.

There is persistent night wheeze or coughing

This is distressing for all concerned. The coughing may go on and on, so that everyone loses sleep. Breathlessness and coughing at night are common in asthmatic children and, if persistent, must be regarded as a sign that the asthma is at least moderately severe and that the *daytime* asthma is not being properly controlled. It will be made worse by an infection.

The doctor's first aim will be to break into the cycle, and this means a short sharp course of steroid tablets. He will also make sure that an adequate dosage of inhaled bronchodilator is administered during the day; this should also be available, when needed, at night. It is quite possible that the child is not using the inhaler correctly or that a spacer would provide a more effective dosage, for example a Nebuhaler or a Volumatic (see page 115).

If regular preventive medicine is not already being used, then this will be needed, in the form of an inhaled steroid, or Intal, to take over when the course of tablet steroid ceases. If inhaled steroids are already being used, then the doctor may decide to increase the dose from twice to four times a day. It is possible that a slow-release bronchodilator, taken last thing at night and effective over eight hours, will help to keep night spasm at bay. This may contain salbutamol (Volmax) or terbutaline (Terbutaline SA) or theophylline (Nuelin SA, Slo-Phylline, etc.). A modern alternative, Salmeterol (Serevent), gives 12-hour protection (see page 96).

When to call the doctor as an emergency

I make no apology for returning to a theme which has already been treated in Chapter Six, 'What to do if things go wrong', on page 136. In childhood asthma, it is the adult who usually has to make this decision; it is essential that he or she can interpret correctly the signs and symptoms which indicate that the attack is so severe that medical help should be sought at once.

Many parents are reluctant to call the doctor, especially at night-time, though this is when the asthmatic is most often at risk. As already explained, the principle to follow is very simple:

WHEN IN DOUBT, SHOUT!

In other words, TELEPHONE IMMEDIATELY. The doctor will not necessarily need to visit, especially if you have worked out a crisis plan in advance and have the appropriate medicines to hand. If the doctor is likely to be delayed, he may decide to call an ambulance – and you yourself should summon one by dialling 999 if you feel that not a second should be lost. When it arrives, you may wish to direct it to a hospital with which you are familiar, and in this case you need to be armed with a special card, to be obtained in advance from that hospital.

The warning signs that asthma has entered a severe and possibly dangerous phase are the same in both child and adult asthma, though the measurements differ. Any one of the following symptoms may be regarded as a warning signal; in practice more than one is likely to appear at the same time.

A severe attack

○ **Breathing rate**. If higher than 50 a minute in a child under five years and higher than 40 a minute in a child over five years, the attack is severe.
○ **Strained breathing**. This is shown by a pulling in of the chest near the neck as extra muscles are brought into play.
○ **Breathing difficulty**, causing problems with eating or drinking.
○ **Speech difficulty**. This clearly suggests a difficulty in breathing; when the child is concentrating entirely on making each breath, then he or she will be silent.
○ **Pulse rate**. This is not easy to take in such circumstances. In children over four, a rate of over 130 a minute would be considered severe.
○ **Vomiting**. This is a sign that so much mucus has accumulated that vomiting is needed to clear it.
○ **A sudden fall in peak flow**. If this falls to one-quarter of the normal daytime or one-quarter of the normal night-time level, the attack is a severe one. A chart illustrating this was given in the last chapter.

Danger signals

○ **Exhaustion**. This is a sign that the attack is very severe. If the child becomes dazed or lapses into unconsciousness, then breathing could cease.
○ **Wheezing may disappear**. This is also a sign of a very severe attack, because the child is not taking in or passing out enough breath to make any noise.

o **A bluish colour**. In light-coloured children a bluish colour may appear in the lips, mouth and nails. This is a sign that there is a serious shortage of oxygen in the blood supply – a danger signal, because the next stage will be a lapse into unconsciousness.

You may have already established which symptoms and signs call for immediate medical attention – preferably well in advance of any of the three DANGER signals appearing. When you call the doctor, you will be advised what medicines to give the child immediately, depending on what is available at the time. They are likely to be the ones indicated in Group D on page 104:

- a high dose of reliever (bronchodilator), via the most efficient means, for example through a spacer or nebulizer. A dry powder inhaler is not likely to help because it needs a strong sharp puff from the patient. When the doctor arrives, he will most probably give salbutamol or terbutaline in a nebulized dose, twenty times the dose provided by just two puffs from an aerosol metered-dose inhaler
- a high dose of tablet steroid (Prednisolone) may be indicated at the same time, as prescribed by the doctor. The effect takes several hours to build

Make a note of the medicines that have been taken (including especially any theophylline preparations) so that the doctor or casualty officer at the hospital will know what is needed additionally.

During and after the severe attack

Since panic is easily communicated to the child and may reinforce the attack, you must remain calm, however alarmed you may feel; there must be a complete absence of fuss. It will probably serve no useful purpose to order the child to breathe more slowly, since the rate of breathing in a severe attack is wholly automatic; instead you should explain that help is on its way and that the medicines may take a little while to bring the attack under control.

The child will adopt the posture which seems most comfortable. The aim, as explained in the last chapter, will be to let the stomach hang forward, to avoid putting pressure on the diaphragm. Avoid feather pillows and dusty cushions. There may be dehydration, due to excessive breathing through the mouth, intense sweating and sometimes vomiting. A glass of water should be at hand. If the child wishes to go to the lavatory, some assistance may be needed. Clothing should be loosened.

Immediately after the attack, the child will be exhausted and will need to rest in order to build up the store of energy that has been depleted. Unless there is a bad viral infection, however, children recover quickly, usually within a couple of days; and it is the parents who will need more time to get over the worry and tension. The doctor will explain how to adjust the treatments so that they revert to normal.

A stay in hospital

It may be prudent, while waiting for medical help to arrive, to prepare your child for a stay in hospital, and you may wish to stay with him or her in the ward for the first night, to provide reassurance in what will seem a strange and frightening environment. If your child is liable to severe attacks and has never previously been inside a hospital, a prior visit to the children's ward when well could be a good plan, so that it seems a normal and friendly place to be in.

Treatment in the hospital to deal with a severe attack is likely to include:

- a bronchodilator given through a nebulizer (terbutaline or salbutamol)
- a short course of steroids at a high dose, given as tablets or as

a slow-release injection

- fluid replacement, through a 'drip'
- oxygen

Relief from the attack will not necessarily be immediate: it may take 2–8 hours to bring it under control. The child will probably be kept in overnight so that progress towards normality can be checked. An X-ray photograph may be taken to make sure there are no lung complications.

In the hospital, the child is the centre of attention; he or she may come home expecting to receive the same four-star treatment. But the parent will be exhausted, keen to catch up on all the neglected chores, and worried that another hospital visit may soon be needed.

Open door admissions

In emergencies it is usually best to get in touch with your G.P. General practices provide round-the-clock emergency cover, either by arrangement with other practices or (in the towns) by using agencies to act for them. The G.P. (or deputy) will decide whether a hospital visit is needed. However, if he is not readily available, it may be wiser to go straight to the hospital. If the child has been admitted frequently then the specialist may arrange an 'open door policy' whereby the child can be taken direct to the hospital without contacting your G.P.

CHAPTER NINE

Schooldays and Holidays

Don't blame the teachers!

Parents often do not realize that few schoolteachers receive any training in how to cope with an asthmatic child. They are denied access to medical records, yet they are supposed to act *in loco parentis*. When there is an attack, the parent may not be available; the teachers may not know who the family doctor is, or what medicine is appropriate.

Parents have only themselves to blame if the teachers believe that asthma is a trivial or nervous illness, or are unaware that the child can play a full part in school activities if the medicines are taken correctly. Teachers act by such rules as they have been given; if told that the 'inhaler' is taken at 2.30 p.m., then they will be reluctant to produce it at any other time.

Each child is different and it is essential that teachers and parents meet and talk over the treatments, with the child present, so that all agree on the right course of action, set down in writing. If this meets with resistance, then a letter from the doctor to the welfare teacher is needed. Better still, the doctor can fill in the *School Treatment Card*, published by the National Asthma Campaign. This specifies both regular and relief treatment.

Practical matters

It must be established that wherever the child goes, the reliever inhaler (Ventolin, Bricanyl, Aerolin) goes too. It will not help if locked in the school cupboard when an attack takes place on a football pitch half a mile away. The preventive use of an inhaler before exercise should be made known to the staff (Intal, or the reliever inhaler).

Make sure that the school has spare inhalers and that your notes make clear which is which ('the blue one is used to relieve an attack; the brown one only for prevention'). No harm will result if another child uses the inhaler in play. The Autohaler and powder inhalers will prevent a game of 'squirts': they fire only when there is an in-drawing of breath.

Teachers are usually aware that they should stay with a child during an attack or a visit to hospital, until the parent arrives. They may not be aware of the need to loosen clothing and the position a child prefers during an attack (see page 141).

The changing role of the school nurse

School nurses have received three years' nursing training. They administer to children, parents and teachers, and in some instances to doctors if the treatment needs to be changed. The nurse has a number of roles, the first of which is to identify any special needs. The second role is to make sure that the condition is understood by *all* the children and teachers, so that the child is not stigmatized or bullied. This is especially a problem with teenagers, who resent being labelled as 'different'. The Asthma Training Centre has produced a training manual for teachers.

The nurse's third task is to make sure that each school has both a school asthma policy and an Asthma Plan which will establish for each child with asthma the correct procedures. The National Asthma Campaign in the U.K. has produced a useful teachers' pack which contains a Policy Statement.

The fourth objective is to work alongside teachers in education. Health Education is not part of the present school curriculum in the U.K., but can be incorporated into it (for example when tackling science). The nurse should also initiate *health promotion*, so that children learn how to say 'no' to cigarettes and 'yes' to exercise.

A fifth objective should be to make sure that the children with asthma are not constantly exposed to potted plants (moulds) or animals (hamsters' urine contains a powerful allergen).

Parents involved in teaching

Some nurses have set up 'puff clubs'; these meet at three o'clock, when the parents arrive to collect their children, and have discussions about treatment. They may bring in the local pharmacist.

Efforts are being made, for example by local branches of the National Asthma Campaign, to address school classes (helped by a film), so that asthma can be explained to all the children. On these occasions the asthmatic children have much to contribute, for example being asked to show the others how well they use their inhalers. Bringing asthma into the open helps to reduce shyness and bullying and may prevent a tragic case such as that of the little girl who died with an inhaler unused in her pocket. When talking to school classes I distribute drinking straws and invite all present to try to breathe through the straws after they have been bent and restricted.

Sport, games and gym

Exercise is one of the ways in which children keep healthy; and it contributes to growth. It is in dream sleep and in exercise that hormones are released which promote normal growth. Taking part in games and sport can improve a child's self-confidence – but only if he or she is able to compete on equal terms with other children.

Most children with asthma become wheezy as a result of

exercise; this is, after all, one of the signs that doctors look for when they diagnose the illness. Typically, the shortage of breath takes place when the child pauses to rest (see page 59) and the attack can last for half an hour or longer.

Teachers should understand that all but the most severely asthmatic children can play a full part in gym, games and sports – but only if certain procedures are followed:

- the child takes an inhaled dose of Intal immediately before the exercise starts, or a dose of Ventolin or Bricanyl a few minutes beforehand (or both)
- extra puffs of Ventolin or Bricanyl may be needed at half time – but this should suggest that better routine *preventive* treatment is needed
- if a peak flow meter (see page 143) is available, this can be used to check that the breathing is up to best level
- warm-up exercises in short bursts help to prepare the lungs for the more strenuous activity that is to follow

Swim groups have been formed

Swimming is so good for asthmatic children that special swim groups have been formed in many parts of the U.K., often in association with local branches of the National Asthma Campaign. There are very good reasons why swimming is ideal exercise for many asthmatic children:

- the body is supported by the water so that less oxygen is needed to carry out movements than in any other form of exercise
- the warm, humid atmosphere of the indoor pool mimics the warm, humid air that is delivered by the upper to the lower respiratory system
- the exercises can be adjusted to the child's condition, and supervision by trained instructors can be provided
- parents and non-asthmatic brothers and sisters can also join in

Some children find that chlorine can trigger an attack; some pools use ozone instead, and this too can cause wheeziness. In any case it is sensible to check with the peak flow meter that the asthma is under control before the swim and to give a preventive dose of Intal or inhaled bronchodilator beforehand. Swimming can restore sagging self-confidence. Picture a child who was described to me by a swim group instructor as not only severely asthmatic but also seen by those 'nearest and dearest' as a 'wimp', a born loser in every department of school life. His father in particular, a soldier who revered physical prowess, seemed to despise and reject him. However, the child decided to take up swimming; as a result he gradually grew stronger. After a couple of years he became the best swimmer in the school. In the following year, the school won the League Championship; he was now a hero to friends and family alike.

The international swimmer, Adrian Moorhouse, had asthma at an early age, and in his teens this interfered with games and running. A chest specialist persuaded him to persevere with swimming – which he did to such good effect that he won a gold medal in the Commonwealth Games, and again at the Seoul Olympics. He has written: 'I don't think that asthma has interfered with my ambition at all, because I haven't let it. I just keep on training. I suppose it made me more determined, because at school I was never going to get into the athletics or rugby team.'

How physiotherapists can help children

In children with asthma the chest muscles are well developed and stronger than in normal children, so special exercises for these muscles are not needed. But there are other ways in which the physiotherapist can help, such as teaching children how to breathe in a more relaxed way, and these are described in Chapter Three, which deals with exercise as a trigger. Very occasionally children get into problems because mucus plugs form in the airways and this can cause the lung beyond the affected area to collapse. The physiotherapist can expand this area, after treatment with appropriate medicines.

Exercise should be imaginative, dynamic, interesting, enjoyable, varied and accessible, and without adverse effects, if it is to become habitual. Physiotherapists are great communicators and can help satisfy these demands.

o Particular care should be taken in windy, cold or damp weather to avoid exercise which is prolonged and which also (like cross-country running) involves the whole body. At my school these runs were known as 'sweats', but they were in reality 'threats'.

o It may be easier to cope with a position on the games field which involves short bursts of running rather than continual motion: in defence rather than galloping up and down as an attacker. But goalkeeping may be seen as a stigma.

o In highly competitive sports the relievers and preventers may be used from inhalers, but not as tablets or injections. Inhaled steroids may not be used in cycle races.

o There are a few sports which your doctor may advise should be avoided. These may conceivably include scuba diving, sky diving and bungee jumping, none of which existed in my youth! On the other hand, the National Asthma Campaign combines with the Eczema Society to run activity holidays for teenagers, who find they can enjoy the most strenuous pursuits, under supervision.

Those dreaded exams

Although bookish, I used to dread exams because they always coincided with the peak time for pollen asthma and hay fever. The questions swam in a watery blur, the anti-histamines used in those days caused drowsiness, and non-selective relievers added to the mood of depression!

Nowadays, preventive medicine can be taken for both asthma (page 97) and hay fever (page 226). If in any doubt, consult your doctor well before the exams are due and keep the peak flow chart up to date. A doctor's letter to the examining board, in advance of the exams, could help in the case of a borderline result. If severe attacks of asthma, or hay fever, are likely, then a course of Prednisolone is a useful standby, to begin a few days beforehand; alternatively, a slow-release steroid injection (Kenalog) can be used. Relaxation exercises may reduce the stress. When the great day arrives, avoid sitting next to an open window.

Advice for child minders

Many parents are working when their children are young and have to find someone to look after them. This can be difficult if a child has asthma. The choice lies between engaging a child-minder or nanny and dropping the child at a day nursery, play-group or nursery school. It is simple common sense to make sure that the minders know how to cope.

The National Asthma Campaign has compiled a short check-list:

- will people be smoking near your child?
- are there any pets to consider?
- will weaning, or food allergy, be taken seriously?
- will the carers give your child medication if needed?
- do they know what to do if there is an asthma attack?
- can they get in touch with you, or a doctor, quickly?
- is the child-care worker registered with the local authority?

As with schoolchildren, it is essential to leave clearly written instructions with the carers. A National Asthma Campaign School Card can be used.

'We do like to be beside the sea!'

In the past, the annual family holiday, nothing more adventurous than a fortnight spent among the seaside rock-pools with a shrimping net, was preceded by weeks of excited and meticulous preparation. Nowadays we fly half-way round the world with the minimum of plans, and young people especially are likely to dash off and leave their medicines behind. This is a mistake, since no country is free from asthma, whether it is hot and humid, dry and dusty or cold and windy. Although the house dust mite is present in fewer numbers above 1,400 metres and is not to be found above the snow line (2,000 metres), mountain air is cooler and drier and contains much less oxygen than you are used to at home. You may therefore need to increase the dosage of preventive medicines when you are on holiday, preferably starting to do so a few days before leaving.

My worst attacks have tended to take place away from home, probably because I encountered new triggers. So relievers, preventers and the peak flow meter should all find a place in your pack, preferably in the hand luggage, even if you are going away for just a weekend. Tablet steroids should be included if prescribed.

In the aircraft, all kinds of inhalers can be used, and they will not alarm the Customs security men. However, warn the carrier in advance if you may wish to use your nebulizer in the aircraft. Few airlines carry them and a large-volume spacer can be just as effective, since it can be used to dispense multiple doses of a relieving medicine.

If travelling to a pleasant climate, you may be tempted to stop using your preventer (Intal, Becotide, Filair, Flixotide or Pulmicort). I did just this in warm, dry, aromatic Provence. Two weeks after returning to cool, wet, polluted London, I ended up in Ward Five West with severe asthma: my guard had slipped and inflammation of the airways had been allowed to set in at a higher level.

In an emergency

You may worry about what to do in an emergency. As explained on page 138, you can take a reliever, such as Ventolin or Bricanyl, repeatedly (up to 30 puffs, separated by 15 seconds between each puff, and preferably from a spacer). At the same time a course of Prednisolone *acute saver* tablets will reinforce the routine preventive medicine taken from an inhaler.

As a precaution, if you are planning to take a holiday away from home, but still in your own country, you can register in advance with a local G.P. In an emergency you can go straight to the Out-patients Department in the local hospital. When travelling abroad, check with the hotel information desk, or courier, where medical help may be obtained.

Modern medicines are available in all the English-speaking countries and in Europe. They are best asked for by their generic name (e.g. salbutamol rather than Ventolin). In the U.S.A. and Canada, theophylline is the most widely used reliever. If you use theophylline, do not allow a foreign doctor to add the antibiotic erythromycine to the prescription. In countries which are both hot and humid, Rotacaps and Spincaps may not work properly, so an aerosol inhaler could be preferable. If in any doubt whether a medicine will be available locally, ring the Medical Information Department of the drug company whose name appears on the pack (see Useful Addresses, page 284).

Finally, if you are planning to travel anywhere overseas, it is wise to take out adequate private health insurance.

CHAPTER TEN

Living with Adult Asthma

The changing pattern of asthma

In early adult life asthma is likely to diminish, to the extent that about 80 per cent of those whose asthma started in childhood achieve a complete recovery at this time. As they pass into middle age and beyond, half of these experience no further trouble, but half have a relapse. Asthma can start at any age, and late-onset asthma is likely to be the kind that persists.

As we grow older, the allergic triggers become less important; the non-allergic irritants, such as virus infections, dry and cold air, and pollutants, such as industrial fumes and cigarette smoke, take over as the most common immediate causes of asthma. When asthma appears for the first time in older people who have had no previous experience of it, there may be no response to the skin prick tests which reveal atopy (allergy).

Adults are better able to monitor their own illness and adjust the treatment. They have more control over the environment at home. They can more easily talk to the doctor about treatment and discover what the medicines are supposed to achieve. On the debit side, asthma in adults can affect earning capacity. There is the special problem of 'occupational asthma' caused by the materials handled, and adults are often affected by the ventilating and air-conditioning systems used in windowless offices. These can accumulate asthma-provoking bacteria, moulds and pollen grains and eject them into the office atmosphere. In some offices, infections spread like wildfire; and the journey to work by public transport presents its own challenge to the adult with asthma.

After a time, we tend to forget what a normal airway feels like. In order to avoid undue exertion or exposure to triggers such as cold air, we adapt life to suit the asthma on a permanent basis. In 1978 the results of a trial were reported, in which the patients' assessment of their asthma was compared with an objective assessment obtained from peak flow readings. It was found that the asthma was nearly always worse than the patient realized – the reverse of what had been generally supposed.

How to recognize the degree of severity

This was covered in Chapter Six and also in relation to children. Adults who are interested in their own asthma may wish to gather all the threads together and consider the progress of an unchecked asthma attack not only in terms of symptoms but also taking into account the physiology, the changes in the breathing tubes and the readings from various tests.

This is set out in the accompanying table, which assumes that no corrective treatment has been given. The aim of the treatment is always to break into the cycle and arrest the downward slide in peak flow well short of the danger level.

The doctor's aim when treating someone with severe and persistent asthma will be to prevent the peak flow from dropping below 'B', and then to lift it to a higher level, closer to the best level, 'A', using preventive medicine (see Fig. 30).

We looked at this kind of treatment in Chapter Six when considering the case of the child Anthony. Adult medication proceeds along the same lines. The rate of improvement will depend on whether treatment starts at 'B', 'C' or 'D' on the severity scale shown in Fig. 30. It can be disappointingly slow and gradual, but in the end perseverance pays.

Type of asthma	*Inflammation*	*Changes in the breathing*	*Symptoms*	*Tests tubes*
mild, episodic	reversible	none, except muscle spasm which reverses	none between the episodes	peak flow returns to normal between the episodes
mild, persistent	permanent	smooth muscle thickens the inner lining becomes leaky; so do mast cells inflammatory cells invade from the blood supply	cough (maybe)	airways narrow if given a histamine challenge and this is a sign of bronchial hyper-responsiveness (BHR)
severe, persistent with acute episodes	permanent	smooth muscle constricts swelling of the tissues increased discharge of mucus ↓	wheeze tight chest cough breathlessness	peak flow depressed below normal readings and below the levels at which symptoms are experienced BHR increases: less histamine needed to produce a 20 per cent drop in peak flow
danger level reached	severe	disorganized ↓ very poor supply of oxygen	very rapid breathing leading to coma	peak flow right down, below 60 per cent of best level

The degrees of severity which are possible in untreated persistent asthma (adapted from A. J. Woolcock, in *European Journal of Respiratory Diseases*, Vol. 69, 1986)

It is assumed that the airways are continually exposed to an assortment of triggers which serve to reinforce the asthmatic response and that no medicines are taken.

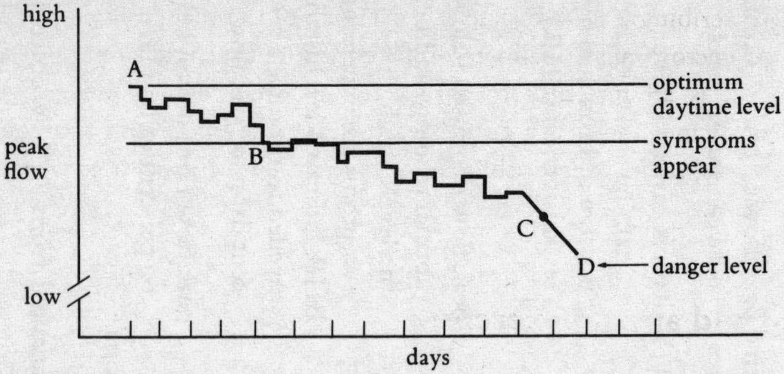

Fig. 30. A slow slide

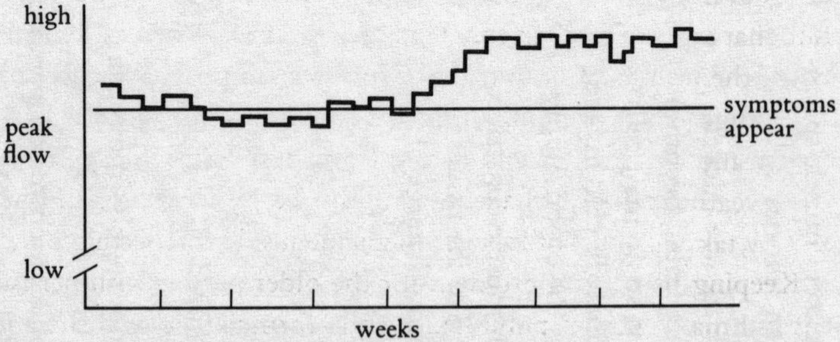

Fig. 31. Successful treatment

The medicines used in adult asthma

The same medicines are used as are appropriate in children: the complete range of bronchodilators and the anti-inflammatory steroids. The anti-allergic drugs (Intal and Zaditen) tend to be used less, since allergy plays a smaller part in adult compared with child asthma. Intal can be used successfully where the adult has a specific allergy, say to cats, combined with a bronchodilator.

If a preventive shield of regular treatment with inhaled steroids is used, then this may be sufficient to prevent night asthma and early-morning wheezes. If these persist, the doctor may consider prescribing a slow-release reliever (one of the theophyllines) or a protector (inhaled salmeterol) taken before the night's rest.

It is all too easy to forget to take the regular preventive medicine, and it is a good idea to leave the inhalers in strategic places, such as the washbasin, so as to get into the habit of taking them.

Cold air and exercise

The medicines will need all the help they can get if they are to keep inflammation at bay. In the case of older people, background central heating may be a necessity, at least in the early morning and in the evening, with good ventilation maintained during the day. I find that an even temperature helps a great deal. When away from home the motor car with closed windows can provide a convenient refuge when bringing an attack under control, since it has a heater and an air filter and is free from dust mites. Shopping in cool weather can be a challenge, minimized by wearing a muffler and by taking a puff of reliever medicine just before setting out.

Keeping fit is a real problem for the older person with persistent asthma. A leaflet published by the former Chest, Heart and Stroke Associaton advises us to: 'Take a regular daily walk. Do not shuffle, a longer stride is more economical than a short one. Do not let your family fetch and carry for you when you can do this job for yourself. Do not take a lift if you can manage the stairs.' If outdoor exercise proves impossible, then indoor exercise is an alternative: 'Choose where to exercise. This can be a staircase, taken at a speed which *just* makes you breathless.' For more ideas about exercise, see page 59.

Asthma treatment and osteoporosis

Osteoporosis is a gradual weakening of the bones due to a loss of calcium. It can be painful and the painkillers used can contribute to dizziness. It can occur in women after the menopause, is more likely to occur in smokers and in people who do not take exercise or who do not have a balanced diet with adequate calcium in it.

A regular daily use of tablet steroids, over a long period, can contribute to osteoporosis, and it is sensible to restrict short crisis courses of tablet steroids to no more than ten days at a time, limited to three or four courses a year. Inhaled steroids are not likely to be a cause of osteoporosis, except at very high, continuous doses.

Asthma in the 'Seventh Age'

Shakespeare – or at least Jacques in *As You Like It* – took a gloomy view of the sixth and seventh ages of man, which the poet never lived to enjoy (or endure). Asthma can, if it is severe and persistent, present special difficulties to people who have reached retirement age, especially when other respiratory diseases are also present. C.O.A.D. is an umbrella term for 'chronic obstructive airway disease', including emphysema, chronic bronchitis and pneumoconiosis. These illnesses are non-reversible and the aim is to stabilize them at their current level, using antibiotics to fight infections, and providing additional oxygen from a cylinder or concentrator if breathing is severely restricted.

Asthma is seen by doctors as the reversible element in respiratory disease, but only within limits because for many now in their sixties and seventies it was not well controlled in the early years and as a result the airways have become less 'elastic' over time. Some were given tablet steroids from the 1960s onwards, in large and regular doses, and then became dependent on this form of treatment. The consequences can be severe.

John, now sixty-nine, has both severe asthma and C.O.A.D. As a result of years of use of daily steroid tablets he has developed osteoporosis of the upper spine. This causes great pain, except when lying down. The pain is relieved with an analgesic, but this is probably responsible for attacks of dizziness. Cataracts in both eyes have proved hard to treat, and John no longer watches television with pleasure and has given up his great hobby, easel painting. A third consequence of the tablet steroids is a huge appetite and consequent weight problem, which aggravates both the asthma and the spinal pain.

The lesson to be drawn by younger generations is to take the inhaled steroids, if prescribed, regularly in the earlier years when the asthma is well controlled. It should then be possible to avoid having to use *tablet* steroids in later life, except for short sharp courses which do not cause problems.

Nobody likes taking medicines day in and day out, especially when in old age they multiply as new ailments appear.

Marie, now sixty-five, decided to stop taking regular doses of inhaled steroids for three 'reasons': an aggressive reflexologist had warned her against them; they had made her hoarse; and a diuretic taken for a kidney complaint had in the past led to facial swelling. She was persuaded that none of these was a rational ground for stopping the inhaled steroids.

As explained in Chapter Four, a large-volume spacer will reduce the amount of inhaled steroid that is swallowed if a metered-dose aerosol inhaler is used. At the prescribed doses of inhaled steroid (Becotide, Becloforte, Filair, Flixotide or Pulmicort), none of the more distressing side-effects of tablet steroids will be experienced.

Asthma and your job

The National Asthma Campaign (United Kingdom) commissioned a survey to discover to what extent asthma interferes with work. Nine per cent of workers had been forced to change their job because of asthma; three-quarters had been upset by passive smoking; over half were affected by fumes or dust in the workplace. Four out of ten felt restricted in the type of work they could do.

At a Branch meeting, a lady told us that when she complained about passive smoking at work her employment soon came to an end. A member of the audience advised her to work for one of the big chains that carries out a no-smoking policy throughout the organization. As a guide to employers, the National Asthma Campaign has produced 'Asthma in the Workplace'. This describes the illness and the medicines. The ideal environment is one which enables people with asthma to avoid exposure to stimuli such as cold, smoking, fumes and allergens. Shift working can help people whose asthma is worst in the early morning. Avoid sitting near the office copying machine: it produces ozone when switched on.

Asthma related to work

It has long been known that certain occupations are associated with asthma; one of the earliest to be recognized was bakers' asthma, due to handling flour. Antonio Vivaldi's father was a baker; asthma prevented the young composer from following the family's trade. 'Occupational asthma' in the strict sense is an illness which exists as a result of the work and is a 'prescribed' disease. Compensation for the ill-health can be obtained in the United Kingdom from the Department of Health and Social Security, provided:

- the substance complained of is listed for compensation
- the substance is present at work
- it can be shown by a doctor that your asthma has been caused by sensitivity to this agent

It can be difficult to detect work-related asthma if, as is often the case, the symptoms are experienced not at the workplace but in the evening or at night. One tell-tale sign is that symptoms fade away during the weekend or when on holiday, though it may take a few days for this to happen.

It is rare for the asthma to develop when you first come into contact with the offending substance. It may begin weeks, months or even years later.

The paint sprayer's tale

John Smith worked happily (we may suppose) as a paint sprayer for many years. He had no symptoms of wheeziness until, at the age of fifty, he was introduced to a new paint system which used isocyanates as a hardener. There were warnings on the can, but these were in German. There was a ventilation system at work, but not a very effective one, and when the wind blew from the east it went into reverse.

John Smith became wheezy in the evenings but improved at the weekends. A year later the asthma had become severe. His G.P. referred him to a chest unit and a 'challenge test' using the suspected hardener confirmed that it was to blame.

The prescription? Simply a change of job, though it took a month for the symptoms to fade away.

It may sometimes be possible to replace the offending substance with a safer material. If this is not possible, it may be feasible to close off the equipment or to fit really effective fume-extractors or to wear a mask.

Unfortunately, workers are often reluctant to cause a fuss, and employers tend to become indignant if it is suggested that their process is harmful. Tact is needed by the doctor who investigates. On the other hand, a change of occupation usually results in an end to the problem – unless the asthma is also caused by other triggers encountered outside the workplace. If you continue in the occupation, irreparable damage may result.

It has been established that cigarette smokers are 5–10 times more likely to develop occupational asthma than non-smokers. This is because cigarette smoke damages the thin linings of the airways, which allows the irritating triggers to pass through them. You will recall that in the Barcelona epidemic (see page 72) it was the cigarette smokers who were most at risk. This is also true of workers who dip electrical components into baths of epoxy resins. These and other chemicals with a low molecular weight are highly reactive compounds which can make chemical changes in the airways as well as in the manufacturing process.

Employment	**Agent**
the farming, milling and baking of grain/flour	grain or flour contaminated with grain weevils, mites or fungal spores
the milling and joinery of wood	wood dust (especially Western Red Cedar)
manufacture of 'biological' detergents and antibiotics	dust from enzymes and antibiotics
laboratory work with animals or insects	urine of rats, mice and guinea pigs; locusts
plastics, paints, adhesives and glues	various chemicals (isocyanates, formaldehyde, epoxy resins, acid anhydride)
refining metals	nickel, chromium, cobalt, platinum
electronics	colophony fumes from soldering fluxes
hairdressing	henna and bleaches

All the above are eligible for compensation if asthma results from exposure to the agent.

Claiming compensation

First consult your general practitioner. He may refer you to hospital for special tests. If the doctors support the view that you have occupational asthma, you then apply (in the United Kingdom) to the Department of Social Security (D.S.S.) for Form NI. 237, which you return to them after you have filled it in. If they decide you are eligible, they will ask you to attend for examination by two doctors; eventually if the D.S.S. supports your claim, they will decide on the level of disablement. You may appeal against an adverse decision to a tribunal.

The list of eligible employments on page 206 is not exhaustive and is included to illustrate the kind of agents that may be responsible for 'occupational asthma'.

CHAPTER ELEVEN

Living with Food Allergy

Is this a common cause of asthma?

At present it is popularly believed that a whole range of illnesses can be ascribed to food allergy. As far as asthma is concerned, the verdict is a mixed one. The experts tell us that food is a much less common trigger for asthma than allergens (such as house dust mite) or irritants (such as infections). On the other hand, it has been established at the Hammersmith Hospital in London that in children with a family history of asthma (especially among children of Indian parentage), the 'hyper-responsiveness' of their breathing tubes can be heightened by some foods in common use.

Food allergy can at times be an immediate and dramatic event. There may be a swelling of the lips and tongue, or an itchy rash, or headache, or pains in the stomach. More rarely, there can be coughing and wheezing. The remedy, where a single food is thought to be responsible, is simply to avoid that food in the future.

An allergic reaction to food may be delayed. This happens when it is caused, not by the food in its ingested state, but by the products which result when we digest it. This makes detection much more difficult.

The gut is where the allergic reaction to food starts. The offending food antigen is able to penetrate the thin skin (**epithelium**) and so enter the intestine and become absorbed in the bloodstream. The immune system recognizes the intruding antigen. In 'normal' people, no further action takes place. But in people who are 'atopic', there may be a vigorous response, even if the invader is no more harmful than the white of an egg. IgE antibodies are produced and attach to the local mast cells and basophils. These release various chemicals, such as histamine; among the many possible responses, a shortage of breath may occur due to a constriction of the breathing tubes.

Any naturally derived food can cause an allergic response, but it is the protein or carbohydrate component which provides the antigen. In children, the foods most commonly responsible are citrus fruits, apples, tomatoes, milk, white of egg, fish (especially shellfish), nuts (for example, peanut butter), chocolate, wheat products and yeasts (such as Marmite), peas, and many spices including ginger in biscuits. As the food-allergic child grows older, so the symptoms become less frequent, and most foods are well tolerated. The exceptions are egg white, fish and nuts, which may continue to produce reactions. Reactions to milk are mostly limited to early infancy.

Food intolerance caused by additives

Food may lead to asthmatic symptoms even when no allergic mechanism is involved; in this case there is a direct, irritating effect; for example, sodium metabisulphate is widely used as a preservative in soft drinks. As soon as the child takes a drink from the can or bottle there is a fit of coughing or wheeze. Mineral water does not produce this reaction.

The supermarket chains are well aware that many of their customers are concerned about food additives. Safeway Food Stores employ a Nutrition Advisory Service, and they have produced free booklets on additives. Booklet No. 1 explains why they are used:

- to enable the food to be prepared more easily
- to make it taste or look better
- to prevent it going stale
- to preserve the nourishment

It seems that the range of additives is vast. The booklet describes the role (among others) of anti-oxidants, preservatives, bulking agents, emulsifiers, crisping agents, stabilizers, thickening agents, sweeteners, flavours, colours and added nutrients. Many of these are both natural and harmless. Their second booklet explains what the E.E.C. codes ('E' numbers) represent. It also puts a star against those additives which may, in sensitive individuals, cause adverse reactions such as asthma.

The food *colour* which is of greatest importance to asthmatics is the yellow Azo dye, tartrazine (E 102). This turns up in syrups and soft drinks, in cakes, biscuits and puddings, in sauces and confectionery, in packet snacks, toppings and pickles. It is also used in medicines to make them yellow, green or orange.

The food *preservative* which causes most trouble in sensitive individuals is the one already mentioned: sodium metabisulphate (E 223 and E 224). This breaks down into the irritating gas, sulphur dioxide. It is not a natural substance, and it is used in acidic foods to prevent bacteria growing, to preserve the colour and to maintain Vitamin C. Avoiding this preservative is not easy, since it is added to beverages, dried fruits and vegetables, sausages, fresh prawns, fruit yoghurt, salad dressings, toppings, jams and flavouring essences.

Peanuts are well known to be dangerous to those few people who are extra sensitive to them. What is less well known is that some infant milk preparations contain vegetable oil derived from peanuts, and there may be traces of peanut protein in some Vitamin D formulations. An article in the *Lancet* (29 May 1993) suggests that this may be responsible for the increase in peanut sensitivity seen in children.

Additives in drinks

Alcohol does not interfere with the medicines used in asthma. However, it may itself be a trigger for wheeziness. This may be caused by the alcohol, or by preservatives, or by yeast used in fermentation, or by flavours added from fruits.

Wines are very complex and contain many potentially allergenic substances. Some sensitive people can tolerate expensive vintage wines better than the cheaper ones; others fare better with 'plonk'! Aldehydes appear in red wine (they give you headaches) but not in white wine. The preservative sodium metabisulphate is used in wines, along with salicylates, which can also act as a trigger. They are not declared on the labels. Champagne contains yeasts, and whisky and gin have added natural flavours which can cause wheeziness.

Beers and ciders also contain preservatives, though in smaller amounts when they are canned. Some drinks, for example Coca Cola, can also cause asthma by virtue of their acidity.

Equally hard to pin down are the natural products which can cause asthma in infants and which are used as carriers for flavourings. Examples include whey powder, dried skimmed milk and lactose. None of these has to be declared on the contents label.

Is salt to blame?

There is one additive that has been used since ancient times, at least among those tribes that abandoned the nomadic life and took up agriculture: salt. It has recently been suggested that there may be a link between a high intake of salt and a susceptibility to asthma. At a conference, Dr Peter Burney showed two maps of the English counties: the first was shaded to represent the local death-rate from asthma, and the second to show the average purchases of salt in all forms, including convenience foods which contain it. The two maps seemed to be almost identical. Both salt intake and the asthma death-rate were highest in the South-East and in the South. Could this be connected with the fact that in these areas there is a greater consumption of convenience foods? Here we enter the realms of conjecture, and more work will be needed before salt is either cleared of suspicion or finally incriminated. Low sodium salt is available at good health food shops.

Should people with asthma avoid certain foods?

This is a matter for debate among specialists. Patients' own reports of food intolerance have often been exaggerated. On the other hand, the interval between the meal and the appearance of the symptoms varies a good deal, so that genuine links reported by patients may be misbelieved. There are challenge tests, but these are suspect.

According to scientists reporting to the European Community, allergic reactions to foods such as milk, fish and nuts affect about 1 per cent of the population, or about 10 per cent of people who are atopic. They calculate that food additives affect only one-fifth of 1 per cent. About one child in 1,000 is sensitive to tartrazine and, for most people, additives are harmless.

A diet based on fresh foods is a sensible alternative to one based on prepared foods, if these are suspected. And if in any case the patient's asthma is well controlled by the use of preventive medicines, then the wheeziness due to food or food additives is likely to be avoided at the same time.

Patients who react strongly to foods usually do so within a few minutes; if additives are suspected, the packet will list them (or most of them!) so that they can be identified. At Guy's Hospital in London, Professor Lessof set up a National Data Bank which shows the components of the prepared foods in daily use, and your doctor can refer to this if in doubt.

Exclusion diets

These are used, under medical supervision, where the asthma is severe and the connection with a particular food is not obvious. There are two kinds of exclusion diet. The first is one in which a single food or ingredient is suspected. It is excluded from the diet for a period; peak flow readings are taken and these can show whether exclusion produced an improvement.

The second kind of exclusion diet is one where no single food is suspected. All foods are excluded from the diet except for a few which rarely cause allergic symptoms. Then foods are reintroduced, one by one. Peak flow readings are recorded and will be depressed when a harmful food is added. This can then be avoided in the future.

If a special diet is continued for a long period, the patient may suffer from a lack of essential nutrients. In children this could restrict growth; for example, there may be a loss of zinc and calcium, of total proteins and of Vitamin D.

Is breast feeding desirable?

The latest evidence suggests that mother's milk does give some protection against the development of an atopic illness and, surprisingly, diminishes any extra risk which might otherwise arise from the mother herself being atopic. The small amounts of antigen present in formulas based on cow's milk can provoke an allergic response. Breast feeding can also reduce the risk of virus infections. For the first three months, the mother's consumption of cow's milk should be reduced but not eliminated, because that would deprive mother and child of essential calcium. In these early days the mother should also avoid the kind of foods that can cause reactions: fish, nuts and cereals, especially if either or both parents are atopic. Switching to soy milk will make no difference in preventing asthma or other atopic disorders such as eczema; goat's milk is not suitable for young babies, and casein hydrolysate, which is derived from cow's milk, is suitable – but at the same time is foul-tasting and expensive.

A trial is in progress in which the diet of lactating mothers is carefully controlled with the aim of reducing allergy later in the infants' lives. This is described on page 175.

Dieting during pregnancy (for example, in a second pregnancy when the first child has developed asthma) is not only unnecessary but also is to be discouraged, since the mother needs all the nutrients that are available in a balanced diet when she is pregnant.

Asthma and weight problems

Asthmatics notice that their wheeziness gets worse after a heavy meal; this is because a distended stomach presses on the diaphragm. There is another reason for avoiding large meals, if these result in one becoming overweight. This extra weight has to be carried around and this needs extra energy, which the lungs have to provide by supplying extra oxygen. In asthma this supply is limited, so the overweight asthmatic will be at a greater disadvantage than the asthmatic who keeps slim, with or without exercise.

Conclusion

There are various ways in which asthma caused by diet can be reduced or eliminated:

- by identifying and avoiding the offending substance
- by trying out an 'exclusion' diet under strict medical supervision
- by the regular use of preventive medicines taken for asthma due to all manner of triggers, of which food is only one
- breast feeding in infancy, possibly with a special diet for the lactating mother
- avoiding being overweight

As in all asthma treatments, the key to success is trial and observation under the supervision of your doctor, always remembering that a balanced diet promotes health and helps fight asthma.

PART TWO

Living with Hay Fever

CHAPTER TWELVE

Living with Hay Fever

A common illness

As we have seen, the nose is a most efficient dust extractor. It removes most of the unwanted particles that enter, and it does so by creating a turbulence caused by its narrow entrance. This throws the air we breathe against a mucus blanket which lines the cavities and traps the particles. The nose also provides the correct temperature and amount of moisture for the air before it enters the lungs.

About one person in ten complains to the doctor that this mechanism has over-reacted. He or she is told that they have 'rhinitis', which simply means any persistent discharge from the nose. If watery and runny, it is known as 'rhinorrhoea'; if thick and congested, it is referred to as 'catarrh'. 'Hay fever' is the most frequently experienced form of rhinitis, and is both seasonal and due to allergy.

Some patients have rhinitis all the year round ('perennial rhinitis'). This may, like hay fever, be allergic in the strict sense that the triggers also show up on skin prick tests. If one or more of these is positive (for example, to house dust mite) you are said to be 'atopic'. On the other hand the discharge may be caused by irritants which do not show up on the skin tests, in which case you have 'non-atopic rhinitis'. Anyone who gets frequent head 'colds' in winter should ask the doctor whether these ought to be regarded as rhinitis and treated as such.

In the ten-year period to 1981, consultations for rhinitis and for asthma doubled, which suggests that airborne pollutants have increased. Among boys rhinitis is most common when they are aged between five and fifteen. Among girls, it is the fifteen-to-twenty age-group that suffers most. Rhinitis is particularly common among people with asthma. In half the sufferers, it disappears – and, for some obscure reason, this often follows a particularly bad year. In most cases it lessens as we grow older and our immune responses become weaker.

What does it feel like?

The symptoms range from a few itchy sneezes while walking to work to something very like a fever, though the temperature stays normal. It is like having a head cold in its most distressing phase, with the added torment of intense irritation, as if a thousand tiny needles were at work in your eyes and nose. You feel as if your head is about to explode. There are fever-like shivers. Your handkerchief quickly soaks and your nose becomes red and sore. The constant sneezing is embarrassing. In addition, there is a feeling of unease and tiredness. Inflammation in the nasal passages can lead to blocked sinuses and, if these become infected, you may lose your sense of smell and have severe pains in the face. In childhood it is especially unfortunate that hay fever reaches a peak during the June examinations, diminishing both concentration and self-confidence. When you have severe hay fever, you want to be left alone, whether child or adult.

In more clinical terms, these symptoms may be summarized as:

- in the nose: 'rhinitis': a copious discharge of runny or congested mucus; sneezing, soreness, needle-sharp irritation and inflammation. Blockage is caused not by the mucus but by an increase in the flow of blood, leading to a swelling in the tissues. Pain in the face shows that the sinuses are blocked. There may be headaches and disturbed sleep. Children wipe their itchy noses with the palms of their hands, leading to a characteristic crease

- in the eyes: 'conjunctivitis'. The eyes become intensely itchy, red and swollen. Particles accumulate in the corners, causing more itching, and they are removed by rubbing, which brings some temporary relief
- in the throat: 'pharyngitis'. This too is itchy and sore and, at the height of the pollen season, there is a tendency to cough and wheeze
- in the ears there may be deafness in children under seven, which often goes unrecognized

In my recollection of childhood, hay fever and asthma were never equally severe on the same day. Sunny weather released the pollens and made me sneeze; damp weather switched off the pollens and turned on the asthma instead. An explanation for this is given on page 42.

What are the triggers?

The triggers for 'hay fever' are of course seasonal, but rhinitis can occur all the year round. The seasonal triggers are the ones already described for asthma in Chapter Three. They can be summarized as:

- pollens from trees (especially silver birch in April and May)
- pollens from grasses (especially timothy, rye and other meadow grasses from the end of May to the end of July)
- pollens from weeds. These cause little trouble in the U.K.; in the U.S.A., ragwort is a major source of allergy
- pollens and scents from flowers and shrubs (according to the individual flowering season)
- mould spores released by fungi (from ripe crops of wheat, oats and barley, from forests, and in old damp houses, from July to October)

If your symptoms start in the spring, you are probably allergic to pollens from trees. If you have allergic rhinitis in the autumn, then moulds should be suspected. Ornamental flowers in the garden are pollinated mainly by insects and their heavier pollen grains do not travel very far, though they can be a problem when brought into the house and placed by the bedside. The grasses, on the other hand, produce pollen which is wind-pollinated and can be carried for hundreds of miles, descending at last on cities as well as on farmland.

All-year-round triggers include the ones already described in Chapter Three with suggestions as to how they may be avoided; not only pollens but also the house dust mite (especially from late autumn) and horses and furry pets. (Food allergy is not thought to be a common cause of allergic rhinitis.)

Non-allergic rhinitis can also occur all the year round, and the triggers include:

- air pollution (exhaust fumes, cigarette smoke, perfumes, nitrous and sulphur dioxide from the burning of fossil fuels, smoke from a wood fire or frying food). At high concentrations exhaust fumes can destroy the cilia and cause nasal membranes to become leaky to irritants in general
- the nose may run more when you take a hot drink or soup, and alcohol increases the flow of blood through the nose and makes it feel stuffy
- climate and temperature play a part, but this varies from one person to the next. Extremes should be avoided: both the very dry air caused by central heating set at too high a level and a very humid climate
- women with rhinitis tend to feel worse when they are pregnant or taking oral contraceptives. Some women have rhinitis only when they are pregnant
- salicylates (not only in aspirin but also present in cheap wines) can cause rhinitis

Why do some people suffer from allergic rhinitis?

The short answer is that they are over-sensitive to triggers such as pollens in their nasal passages. There are two distinct stages; to be successful, preventive treatment should precede the first stage.

Stage one

Pollen is trapped in the mucus lining of the nose. The chemicals from the pollen manage to penetrate the lining and reach white blood cells (lymphocytes) which circulate in the bloodstream. These lymphocytes respond by producing IgE antibodies in large numbers. In time, these manage to attach themselves to mast cells and, by so doing, form 'receptors' so that the mast cells are primed and ready for the next stage, like a pistol waiting to be discharged. At the same time, these mast cells manage to escape through the thin epithelium which lines the nasal passages.

Stage two

More pollen arrives, perhaps a few weeks later, and cross-links those IgE receptors in the manner described in Chapter Two on page 25. This causes an explosion of the mast cells, so that they shoot out chemicals such as histamine in great quantities. These chemicals produce the symptoms of hay fever already described.

It seems that in 'normal' people the immune mechanism identifies the particles we breathe by means of 'T-cells'. If the particles are harmful, for example germs and viruses, they encourage the lymphocytes to form all those IgE antibodies. If on the other hand the intruders are quite harmless, like pollen grains and house dust particles, then the T-cells act instead as suppressors and no IgE antibodies are formed. It has been suggested that in allergic (atopic) individuals, the T-cells can promote the production of IgE but have no power to suppress it; so IgE is made inappropriately in response to pollen grains, possibly through a genetic defect.

It is also possible that virus infections, so common in early childhood, and early exposure to the passive inhalation of tobacco smoke contribute to this malfunction. Once the level of IgE antibody circulating everywhere goes up, it stays at a high level so the mast cells are primed to respond to the next invasion of pollen grains and other atopic triggers.

Professor Robert Davies of St Bartholomew's Hospital, London, has described the fruits of recent research. Medical students who were atopic allowed tiny extracts to be taken from the tissues of their nostrils after pollen had been sprayed up them. The tissue extracts are stained so as to allow examination under the powerful electron microscope. This procedure is repeated at intervals.

This research has shown that as the hay fever season advances the mast cells increase eightfold and the proportion of mast cells which rise to the inner surface increases fourfold. This means that early in the pollen season the mast cells increase 32 times at the sites where they can respond most readily to the invading allergens.

Implications for treatment

This research, partly funded by the National Asthma Campaign, has three important implications for sufferers:

o When trying to block the mast cells with the preventive medical treatments described below, do not wait until the peak pollen season arrives in June but start early in May. Most sufferers first notice symptoms when the official pollen count is published for the first time. They should delay no longer. If the spring is cooler or drier than usual, the pollen season will be earlier. If you are sensitive to tree pollens, you have to start in March.

o The main purpose of treatment will be to reduce inflammation in the air passages, and for this purpose the preferred method will be to use corticosteroids.

o If you manage to block one allergen (say, pollen) you will stand a good chance of resisting all the others (dust, moulds, dander) and there will be less of a risk that rhinitis will continue into the autumn and winter.

The pollen count

In the United Kingdom this is measured at sites around the country under the auspices of the National Pollen and Hay Fever Bureau at the University of North London. It arrives, rather crudely, at the daily average number of pollen grains in a cubic metre of air: 200 is regarded as 'very high' and below 50 as 'low'. One of the highest counts ever in Central London was 870, recorded on 17 June 1964. In 1993 the numbers of people who went to their doctors with symptoms increased by five times. Hay fever sufferers are sensitive to quite low counts, especially when 'primed', and should rely on their own judgement as to how they will respond, assisted by the weather forecast.

The amount of pollen released varies not only from day to day but even from hour to hour. On sunny days with a light wind it rises high into the air on the warm up-currents and descends in the late afternoon, so that high counts are often seen from 5 p.m. to 6 p.m. It is a good plan to keep the windows shut during peak pollen times. On cool damp days, only a little pollen is released.

Managing hay fever successfully

Can you take avoiding action? The answer is an emphatic 'YES'. There are four kinds of preventive measures.

o Take preventive medicines every day; you should *start before the pollen season begins* and continue until it ends.

o Stay indoors as much as possible and keep the rooms cool and shaded and the windows shut, especially in the late afternoon and early evening, when the grass is being mown. Mowing the lawn releases millions of pollen grains and mould spores and should be left to someone else to do. (Paving stones might be a sensible long-term alternative.) Wear dark glasses to protect the eyes against dust as well as sunshine. Avoid cigarette smoke. If you are studying or sitting examinations, sit as far as possible from open windows.

o When choosing a holiday, it seems best to go away at the height of the local pollen season if you can. At the seaside, the sea breezes blow on to the land and keep the pollens at bay, but in mountainous country the rising air-currents sweep up the sloping pastures and take the pollens with them. In Scandinavia the grass pollen counts are usually low, but avoid the May flowering of the forests of birch trees. House dust mites do not thrive in the dry air of the Alps, so skiers and walkers can enjoy a temporary respite from rhinitis. When driving, keep the windows shut.

o Desensitization
Desensitization is only appropriate when the symptoms are (a) atopic, (b) really disabling, and (c) have not responded to other treatments. To treat hay fever, pollen extracts are injected before the season starts and continued each season for two or three years. In non-seasonal rhinitis, dust extracts are used (see page 58).

Preventing the symptoms with medicines

A the nose

(Before using a nasal spray, it is a good idea to clear the nose of the accumulated secretions.)

As explained above, you should start to use a *preventive* steroid nasal spray while the mast cells are still in their winter quarters: start early in May (or in March for tree pollen) and use night and morning. Continue until the end of the pollen season, even

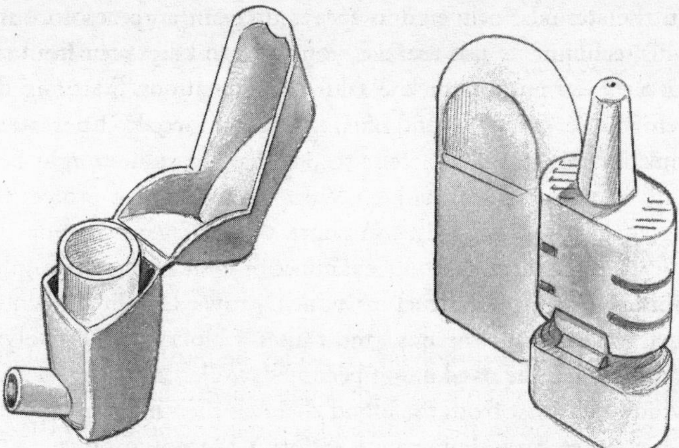

Fig. 32. Beconase and Flixonase sprays

when you have no symptoms. If you adopt this treatment it is unlikely that any nasal symptoms will develop. There are liquid sprays (Beconase Aqueous, Flixonase and Syntaris) and there are aerosols (Beconase and Rhinocort).

A nasal form of sodium cromoglycate, Rynocrom, is used four times a day to supplement the steroids in young people, so as to avoid a high dose when the hay fever is severe. It is available as a powder, a spray and as drops.

If the nose is blocked, use nasal steroid drops. These must be dropped into the nose; the best way to administer them is to lie down on your back on the bed with your head hanging down over the edge of the bed so that the drops can reach the nasal passages. They are taken every day during the pollen season. Brand names are: Bethesol Nasal Drops and Vista-Methasone. A new antihistamine, azelastine (Rhinolast), is available as a nasal spray.

You may start the nasal treatment too late or find that the rhinitis persists into the autumn and winter. In this case a short course of tablet steroid (Prednisolone) may be indicated, taken as three 5mg. tablets each day for two weeks. You can then stabilize on the steroids, delivered as sprays or from an aerosol canister. This technique is also useful if you want to keep your head clear for a special purpose such as taking examinations. Start two days before the special event. An alternative would be a steroid injection (Kenalog).

Nasal polyp

This is a pale-grey structure which grows first in the sinuses, then extends into the nose and causes a blockage. The polyp is caused when the nasal lining becomes swollen and attracts water, which leaks first from the blood channels then from the proteins, which stretch the lining until it forms the polyp or sac. There can be pains in the head, and a persistent drip of mucus into the nose. It can cause bad breath when there is an infection.

The treatment is the same as when dealing with perennial rhinitis, with the possible addition of an antibiotic. A steroid injection (Kenalog) may be considered.

Snoring can be another consequence of a stuffed-up nose, so a course of Beconase could be tried if this creates a social problem!

B the eyes (the eyes have to be treated separately from the nose)

The eyes can be treated with anti-inflammatory eye-drops. Sodium cromoglycate (Opticrom drops) stabilizes the mast cells and is very safe. It has to be used four times a day for both seasonal hay fever and year-round allergic rhinitis. Prednisolone eye drops (Predsol) are always effective; they are taken over a short period under a doctor's supervision.

An alternative is to use one of the newer tablet anti-histamines such as Clarityn, Hismanal, Triludan or Zirtek; they will also reduce symptoms in the nose. A dose is taken once a day and causes very little drowsiness. The few side-effects may include headache, skin rash and an upset bowel.

A short course of tablet steroid (Prednisolone) will also reduce itchiness in the eyes, because it is the same inflammatory mechanism that is at work as in the nasal passages. If injections of corticosone are proposed, the sufferer should be aware that there is a danger of local muscle wasting at the injection site and the possibility of long-term side-effects.

	the nose	the eyes
Steroids		
Aerosol sprays	Beconase (beclomethasone) Rhinocort (budesonide)	
Spray pumps	Beconase Aqueous Flixonase (fluticasone) Rhinolast (azelastine) Syntaris (flunisolide)	
Drops	Bethesol (betamethasone) Vista-Methasone	Predsol (Prednisolone)
Intal (cromoglycate)		
Capsules of powder	Rynacrom	
Drops		Opticrom
Steroid tablets	(Prednisolone)	
Anti-histamine tablets	Clarityn (loratidine) Hismanal* (astemizole) Pollon-Eze* (astemizole) Seldane* (terfenadine) Triludan* (terfenadine) Zirtek (cetirizine)	

The brands used for treating allergic rhinitis

Those marked with an asterisk (*) can be bought over the counter in pharmacies in the U.K. Generic names are given in brackets.

Unsuitable and unusual remedies

Decongestant drops are widely used to treat hay fever – they should be avoided. They are designed to shrink the swollen nasal linings and they do so effectively, so that you feel better. Then there is a rebound and the swelling returns, this time in a more severe form . . . So you take more drops. You end up either being permanently bunged up or the mucus blanket dries and leaves the linings exposed to germs. Thus you pass from an acute phase into a more or less permanent condition, and all this is unnecessary because there are excellent remedies, as have been described.

On a less serious note: in 1881 'Cigars of Joy' provided soothing substances. In 1891, hay fever could 'positively be cured by the Carbolic Smoke Ball'! In 1936, a means was devised of passing radio waves through the head, directed at some obscure region of the brain. In the 1950s, people went on sea-cruises or installed air purifiers. In the 1960s, a school was built underground in the U.S.A. In the early 1980s, a protective helmet, the 'Bubblehead', was advertised and is still available. A 'laminar flow helmet', which was designed for asbestos workers, filters the air and may be useful in the case of some severe occupational allergies.

PART THREE

The Human Response

CHAPTER THIRTEEN

The Human Response

As seen by others

Perhaps the most distressing aspect of asthma and hay fever, when not well controlled, is the way they can mess up ordinary human relationships, the ones everyone else takes for granted. The symptoms are usually concealed so that we can appear to be fit and well and yet be constrained to behave at times as if we are invalids. We (reasonably) decline to take part in activities which to those who are free from these illnesses seem to present no kind of threat. Children, in particular, are under suspicion that they sometimes use their asthma to obtain favours or avoid unpleasant tasks; but this may be a reasonable defence against challenges which they have, in the past, shown that they are unable to overcome. This is especially the case in a society which applauds achievements in sports and games.

A distorting mirror

Whether we like it or not, the way each of us sees our own illness is powerfully affected by the way other people look at it, not only family and friends, and colleagues at work, but even strangers. We are often astonished at the response which casual acquaintances make when the illness is mentioned; they ask us to confirm their belief that the 'illness is due to nerves, isn't it?'. For some reason, hay fever is not popularly ascribed to nerves but to pollens, though the mechanisms are similar! On the other hand, the uninformed response may go to the opposite extreme and suggest that we have a crippling disease which carries a life sentence.

To obtain a detached view of these attitudes, I persuaded a friend who carries out 'group discussions' for commercial purposes to conclude a few sessions with the topic, 'How do you view asthma as an illness?' There were separate groups for adults and for children, and no one had asthma. The views expressed are given here as direct quotations.

Adult manual workers tended to be both realistic and fatalistic:

- 'An asthmatic's lung capacity is a lot lower than a normal person's.'
- 'I have a cousin who was pensioned off at twenty-two because of asthma.'
- 'My step-brother lost his job as a park keeper, just couldn't breathe.'
- 'Most people rate it at three [on a scale of ten] but I rate it at nine.'

White-collar respondents on the other hand came across as rather dismissive:

- 'One of my son's friends gets it, so as soon as he walks through the door we say "Have you got your inhaler?" Really it's up to the individual to control it.'
- 'I've seen kids running around and getting short of breath, but one little squirt and they're as right as rain. I'd have thought in 99 per cent of cases it is only an inconvenience.'
- 'The people I've known with asthma, one puff and they're OK.'

The children were either completely unaware ('Is it the same as hay fever? . . . as eczema?') or concerned and observant:

- 'I used to baby-sit for a child with asthma and it was awful – you think they are going to die in front of you.'
- 'He's like an animal on the football field but all the precautions he takes before, blowing his nose, puffing away, you'd think he wasn't going to last six months.'

- 'They hate people fussing – all those people round her and you could see she wanted them to go away.'
- 'This girl at school almost goes blue because she doesn't want to use the inhaler, so we all shout at her when we see her go like that.'

It is in the schools where the biggest advances in understanding can be made, but this will take place only when the adults have learned more about asthma.

Asthma as seen by parents

The general lack of understanding as to the true nature of asthma bears especially heavily on parents of asthmatic children; I asked two friends with experience of asthma in very young children to describe their worries and frustrations.

> The only two people I had known who had asthma had died from it, so when I was told my baby might be asthmatic I was quite frankly terrified. I did not know where to turn for informed advice. The most that family and friends could offer was a few words of 'Poor you' and 'Oh dear!' and they simply did not want to become involved. Asthma is not nice to talk about, unless there are several asthmatics in the family, and then you get the old wives' tales and the attitude: 'You've just got to put up with it, my dear . . . nothing can be done about it.' It can take a parent a long time to learn how to cope with an asthmatic child. Each parent needs the other's support; it must be very hard indeed for one parent if the other is unsympathetic or simply does not want to know: unfortunately, not an uncommon experience. I know of marriages that have failed because of the strain of coping with asthma.

The second mother's account also stresses the sense of isolation, but this can bring a strengthening of the marriage:

> If they have an asthmatic child, parents have to cope with a feeling of failure. There is the nagging thought that 'if only that chest infection

had been cleared up, asthma would never have developed'. Added to that there is a sort of character assassination by friends who hint that the child is over-indulged and playing up, using the illness to obtain sympathy, a 'typical asthmatic'. In reality there are nerve-racking moments, as when you have to administer a nebulizer and the child is terrified of the noise it makes. Problems with diets (no eggs) means turning up at all the children's parties and this receives adverse comment. Then you have to worry about the non-asthmatic sister or brother who has to compete for the mother's attention and does so by being aggressive. The sad thing is that you can lose a lot of friends through having an asthmatic child . . . but this does bring the family very close together.

Another mother has written: 'When a severe attack occurs I have to go into automatic control in order to be able to cope, and this is followed by complete exhaustion, physically and emotionally, while the child has become quite relaxed and active.'

It is an understatement to say that asthma has its ups and downs. Parents take a year or two to learn how to manage their child's asthma. Everything seems to be well controlled – then, out of the blue, the child has a sudden severe attack for which there seems to be no clear explanation. This is deeply unsettling. The parents feel that they must start all over again, learning how to manage the asthma. As one mother has put it, 'The first dash to Casualty after a long period of relative calm can reduce the parents to the same nervous, unsure, guilty state they were in when the asthma was first diagnosed.'

Over- and under-protection

At a meeting of a self-help group, there was sympathy for the mother who, though aware of the dangers of being either too hard or too soft on her asthmatic daughter, admitted that she tended to swing from one extreme to the other and back again.

Keeping an even balance between the two is not at all easy, especially if you worry about being thought of as 'just another fussy mother'.

Over-protection can, in a small number of children, make the asthma worse. This is shown by the dramatic improvement which can take place when asthmatic children are removed from home tensions for one reason or another.

Parents sometimes feel that their children are only pretending to wheeze, in order to gain attention. Wheezing is a more acceptable way of gaining attention than crying! But the pretend wheeze can physiologically trigger a real attack. A child may 'forget' to use the inhaler, and this produces a genuine wheeze, which gives the same result. It is therefore possible for some families to become caught up in a cycle from which neither parents nor child can escape. This is why a stay in hospital or with relatives can by itself make a child's asthma better. A parent has written:

It is very natural to panic when you see your child struggle for breath . . . No doubt you will resolve to fight against another attack, even another attack occurring. But isolating your child from infection, not allowing the child to take part in strenuous exercise, and not applying discipline lest the emotional upset brings on an attack, is not going to help. The child needs to know that he is as good as his peers, and should not regard himself as 'delicate'.

Parents with an asthmatic child who is strong-willed and assertive face a special kind of challenge, one that has been described by a mother in these words:

Since our third child developed asthma some years ago, as a three-year-old, our family has lurched from crisis to crisis. I was terrified that he would die, because the attacks were dangerously severe, and he has become the centre of our life. After many months his condition was brought under control, although he was ill more often than not. He has a will of iron. No doubt we spoiled him, and family life centred around his needs. As he grew older he became a tyrant, an expert manipulator, insisting on playing football on damp days when it made him ill, and the illness then demanded total attention. My two older children became second-class citizens in our home, selflessly protecting their demanding younger brother.

Finally, I arranged to visit a psychiatrist. He did not blame me but pointed out that, in spite of the attention, our son has felt different and therefore isolated from the rest of the family. We should in future treat him as any other child, showing no more interest in his asthma attacks than we would a cold or sore throat in the other children. If he behaves like a two-year-old he should be treated the way a two-year-old is treated. There would be no more get-well presents . . .

In this situation the young child has taken on too much responsibility, and has suffered from the emotional pressure.

From the child's viewpoint

In a survey published in the U.K. in 1993, four out of ten children with asthma feel panicky, irritated or suffocated when their asthma is at its worst. The same publication reported that asthma made playing with friends difficult.

In my childhood, asthma was thought not to be preventable and, like tuberculosis, to require copious draughts of fresh air, by day and by night. At school, conformity was all-important, and in those days success at games was essential for self-esteem. Failure to shine on windy playing fields tended to make one an 'outsider', and it is hard for children to be cast aside because of their essential nature.

Late maturing can hold back development in all aspects of life, not simply the physical ones. Children inevitably see themselves as being responsible for their illness, unless this misconception can be removed.

Nowadays preventive medicine can allow play to be both normal and natural. Children with asthma can learn to tolerate exercise of increasing severity, provided the steps towards this are gradual. If barred from games, a child may lose a great deal. As Freud wrote; 'Our sense of identity is rooted in our physical being.' Play is essential for the development of all young primates, whether apes or gorillas, or human children. Play stimulates, enables children to feel that they belong, and develops social skills. It provides opportunities for laughter and tears, teaches endurance and tests aspects of personality.

From the adolescent's viewpoint

Adolescence is a difficult time, even without a disability such as asthma. It is a time when self-confidence is put to the test; additionally there are hormonal changes which, in girls, bring with them the monthly cycle, and this can itself influence the ups and downs of asthma.

Teenagers want, above all, to be like – and to be liked by – their companions. They want to be able to join in everything, including games, dances and crowded parties. Any one of these can bring on wheeziness, for example just rushing out into the cold from a disco dance. Teenagers are reluctant to be seen using their inhalers, so they may neglect to do so. As Gerald Scarfe, the cartoonist, severely asthmatic in childhood, mentioned in his autobiographical film: 'I was ashamed of my illness, because it made me feel different.' At times the asthmatic teenager has to stand and watch while others play. On the other hand, some teenagers say they would not like to lose their asthma altogether!

Teenagers attach more importance to good company than to good health. It is as hard to persuade them to give up smoking as to take the medicines prescribed. They do not want to be reminded of these restrictions at a time when they are testing their personality and when their peers are demonstrating what

Professor Milner aptly calls 'fatalistic bravado'. However, G.P.s are seen by teenagers as suitable advisers.

What role can the parents play? Their advice on any topic is unwelcome; it is felt by their teenage children that parents cannot possibly understand the emotional upsets and upheavals. I asked a mother who is at present coping with a teenage asthmatic to provide an answer. She has written:

> I think it is important to see the problem as a whole, and not just from the viewpoint of asthma. When children reach their eleventh or twelfth year we parents should take time to talk to them about the difficulties they will face, explain that they will reject parental advice on many matters and that they will have to be strong and rely on their own code of self-discipline.
>
> Let them begin to manage their own asthma at an early age: ten years old is not too young for some children. Teach them how to use a peak flow meter, how to check whether their inhaler is full or nearly empty, and that they know when to use it. Try to make them understand that asthma is a common illness which they have to accept and learn how to control by themselves so that for most of the time the disadvantages become quite bearable.

There is one aspect of education which may become neglected in the teenage years, in all children, not merely by those with asthma. It is surely unfortunate that the creative abilities, carefully fostered in the primary schools, tend to wither away during adolescence, especially when schools are deprived of funds to devote to the arts. In later life I have derived great consolation from creative pursuits begun in my teens. I talked about this to an asthma group in Chelmsford and a member of the audience agreed emphatically: 'When I am painting I forget about asthma completely.' Crafts taken up in childhood and skills acquired in the teenage years can provide an absorbing interest for a lifetime. As Sir Winston Churchill wrote in *Painting as a Pastime*: 'Painting is a friend who makes no undue demands, excites to no exhausting pursuits, keeps faithful pace even with feeble steps.'

As seen by adults

Since the first edition of this book appeared, surveys have been published which have revealed the way adults' lives are affected by asthma.

In a 1990 survey of 87 asthmatic people between the ages of 16 and 60 in North Staffordshire, a fifth were severely restricted in their activities, and over a half were restricted to some extent. Two-thirds found that exercise caused asthma, and a quarter reported a restriction in activities at work.

'Action Asthma' published a National Asthma Survey which was conducted in the same year. Of the 19,000 respondents in work, half said they had to take some time off work in the last year; 8 per cent had not been able to work at all because of their asthma. Nationally, this will have amounted to about 6 million lost working days, based on the government's data.

In this year again, a study into the Life Quality of Asthmatics showed that nearly 80 per cent found that asthma made some difference to their lifestyles. Most wanted to achieve an improvement in walking, running or generally getting about. A third said they wanted an improvement in sleeping. Some found that their social lives were restricted; they were embarrassed by asthma and by the attitudes of other people to it.

These respondents included many who were prescribed preventive medicine, and this suggests that there is a great gulf between the claims made that modern treatment can enable most people to lead a normal life, and the reality (which tends to be hidden from the doctors).

There is little chance of growing out of asthma which persists into adult life or which starts in middle age. It can appear to the sufferer as a kind of life sentence and it is all too easy to adopt a fatalistic approach and give in too easily, especially if, in the early stages, the treatments are not successful. However, it is not a good idea to adopt a fatalistic approach.

If it is any consolation, my own asthma went out of control at one stage. What should I do? Should I give up my job and move to a more congenial climate? In the event, I pestered the doctors to teach me how the medicines were supposed to work, and I joined the Asthma Society (forerunner of the National Asthma Campaign). After three years of trial and error I learned how to used the medicines more effectively and also how to avoid some of the triggers. As a result, I can now lead an active life, and I draw comfort from the fact that those very severe attacks are now less frequent.

Relatively little has been written by people with asthma about their own illness. Dr Anthony Storr, in his illuminating and extended foreword to Dr Lane's *Asthma the Facts*, gives a personal and moving account of what it is like to experience severe asthma, his dislike of having to take the medicines each day and the adjustments that have to be made to everyday living.

As seen by psychiatrists

Is there an 'asthmatic personality'?

It would not be surprising if people with asthma – at least those with a severe form of the illness – were to develop some neurotic traits and acquire a reputation for being eccentric. But it seems that, by and large, people with asthma are neither more nor less neurotic than the population at large.

In 1970, Dr Andrew Zealley and colleagues in Edinburgh examined the personalities of three groups of people, using standard tests to discover neurotic tendencies. One group was super-normal (they had no neurotic traits); a second group was drawn from people known to be neurotic; the third was composed of 70 asthmatics, selected on a random basis. The asthmatic group emerged as being neither more nor less obsessional, over-sensitive and over-anxious than normal people; in other words, they were mid-way between the two control groups; they were much less neurotic than the neurotic group. Only in one category was their score higher than 'normal': they tended to lack self-confidence. It is hardly a matter for wonder that an illness which strikes at the air supply, at the basis of life itself, and can do so for days on end, should diminish self-confidence.

There is one way in which asthma can interfere directly with ordinary relationships. Some people with asthma, from childhood onwards, tend to talk rapidly and to pause in mid-sentence. If a friend tries to fill in this gap, the asthmatic either subsides completely or overrides the interruption as soon as the missing breath arrives, appearing to be over-assertive but in reality feeling himself to be at a disadvantage.

Is asthma 'psychosomatic'?

Translated into plain English, this question is really asking whether the top brain can directly influence spasm in the airways. There is plenty of evidence in the medical literature that it can do so, by a 'conditioned response'. A very suggestible person may become wheezy when presented with a perfectly formed artificial rose or a picture of a cat – if the equivalent real objects produce this response. Relief from an inhaler may be achieved in some patients, even when an inert substance has been substituted for the active drug. At St Thomas's Hospital in London it was shown that a film depicting horrifying scenes caused reduced peak flow in the asthmatic patients who saw it. This is not surprising: we all become tense when horrified.

Higher centres in the brain can cause the airways to contract through the parasympathetic nervous system, or to relax when stress causes adrenaline to be released. But these asthmatic responses can take place only if the subject has asthma in the first place and it does not prove that asthma is a 'nervous condition'. There are many other triggers which may cause wheeziness, and it is only a minority of people with asthma who can react to 'dummy' allergens.

When reading this section, Dr A. W. Frankland has reminded me that, when lung transplants take place, it is the transplanted lung (with all links to the donor's brain removed) which determines whether the recipient will have asthma. If a lung from a normal person is transplanted into someone who previously had asthma, the asthma will cease. The reverse is also the case: an asthmatic lung will confer asthma on a recipient who was previously free from it.

Can psychotherapy help?

Asthma may be triggered by stress and may itself be a source of profound anxiety. Any doctor who takes the trouble to listen to an asthmatic patient's problems and explain how the illness can be controlled will do much to allay the anxiety. As we shall see, there are sensible ways of relieving stress and dealing with everyday problems.

Psychotherapy in its strict sense can be used to relieve asthma in two kinds of situation. The first is where the asthma is reinforced by a profound, perhaps buried anxiety which, if identified and faced, will disappear and so remove a cause of the asthma. The second is where a patient, perhaps unconsciously, is using the asthma to manipulate another member of the family. If this is brought into the open and recognized, then the symptoms may diminish. Depressive illnesses are treated not with psychotherapy but with the appropriate drugs.

Suffering in silence

A doctor in general practice and trained in psychiatry, after surveying his own patients and those in neighbouring practices, has reported that asthmatics, far from using their illness to demand attention when it is not needed, are generally reluctant to seek help when they should do so. They prefer to manage by themselves. This has led some psychoanalysts to suppose that asthma develops out of conflicts which arose in childhood and are then bottled up, especially conflicts with demanding parents. However, as Dr Storr has pointed out, these conflicts are experienced by all children, so they cannot be responsible for asthma, which is suffered by only a few and is genetic in origin.

Most physical conditions are influenced by stress: headaches are one obvious example, and we can become breathless with excitement. The kind of stress that can contribute to asthma is, according to trained observers, seldom the short sharp stress but is more likely to be the long-drawn-out family row, or continuing worry about exams, or mounting pressures and rising fatigue at work. People vary a great deal in the amount of stress they can handle, and people with asthma vary a good deal in their perception as to how severe their own symptoms are. One is totally disrupted by only mild asthma while another leads a normal life, even though afflicted by asthma which is at times severe.

In later life, there is a tendency to withdraw from the social world when restricted by a disability, so as 'not to be any trouble to anyone', especially if the illness is not understood, or when living alone. I have found that two absorbing interests help to keep the doors open to the outside world. They happen to be easel painting and writing; but *any* creative activity helps.

Four ways of relieving stress

Stress is very common. So is asthma. It is not therefore surprising that it is possible to experience both at the same time. In older children, resentment arising from asthma is likely to be expressed not in words but in aggressive behaviour, such as the slamming of a door in response to a quite reasonable request. This is perfectly natural, and there is no way parents can try to prevent their children from getting upset – nor should they. No one can protect a child (or an adult) from the normal reactions to stress: anger, worry and excitement. Instead:

○ Encourage the child (or adult) to talk about the stress or worry and quite literally 'get it off his chest'. This may require the subtle tactic of referring to your own frustration and asking whether the feelings are shared.
○ If there are family quarrels, try to sort the problem out – with outside help if need be.
○ Encourage the asthmatic to find out which physical stresses can and which cannot be tolerated. When choosing a recreation, sport or career, aim to avoid as many of the stressful situations as possible. Swimming indoors in a heated pool is ideal.
○ Encourage relaxation techniques of any kind. When we are tense, the muscles get tense – including the bronchial muscles. The exercises can be practised from the age of five upwards and should be made enjoyable. As has already been mentioned, swimming is particularly good for asthmatics: it requires controlled breathing; it helps people to relax and 'let off steam', and promotes self-confidence.

A mother has written: 'Parents who do not talk to their children about asthma are doing the child a disservice. Even quite young children with the illness can be reassured if the treatment is explained in simple terms. At the same time, be calm and positive about the illness. Do not allow the child's asthma to take over or transmit any of your worries [about the asthma] to the child.'

The role of the health professionals

The Patients' Charter

In 1992 the U.K. Department of Health amended the Patients'

Charter so as to include ten 'rights'. These are the right

- to receive care on the basis of need, not the ability to pay
- to be registered with a G.P.
- to receive emergency medical care at any time
- to be referred for a second opinion *if you and your G.P.* think this to be desirable
- *to be given a clear explanation* of any treatment proposed, including any risks and alternatives
- to have access to your health records
- to choose whether or not you wish to take part in medical research or student training
- to be given detailed information on local health services, including maximum waiting times
- to be guaranteed admission no later than two years from the day a consultant places you on a waiting list
- to have any complaint about the N.H.S. investigated

In 1993 the National Asthma Campaign published its own Asthma Manifesto, as a guide to patients and health professionals alike. This is set out in full in Chapter Sixteen.

Making friends with your general practitioner

Patients and doctors often have different aims. Some patients expect doctors to work miracles and to 'cure' them. This is not possible with asthma. Given the sense of isolation, and sometimes of despair, patients with a disability such as asthma tend to seek from doctors the kind of moral support that may be lacking elsewhere. It is, however, rare for doctors to be trained in this kind of counselling: they concentrate on physical causes and medicines and do not always want to be involved with all the factors that may contribute to illness in the home. However, they should at least start the consultation by finding out how much you already know about the illness and allow you to explain your problems in your own terms, including any anxieties.*

As far as asthma is concerned, the doctor aims to reduce symptoms and to check progress from time to time. He or she is keen to provide the skills needed for *self*-management and, to this end, to *educate* the patient. But few of us are especially keen or qualified to receive this kind of instruction, beneficial as it may be! There is a limit to what we can take in at any one consultation. When we fail to take the medicines as prescribed, we are labelled 'non-compliant'; but I have suggested (on page 143) that this is a more complex issue than is generally assumed to be the case.

The relationship between doctors and patients is changing. The Guidelines for asthma management are providing a greater uniformity of treatment. Management cards are used increasingly, as described in Chapter Seven. Records of peak flow readings provide a common ground for discussion. Practice nurses are beginning to take over the role of teaching the skills needed to manage asthma successfully. Systems of auditing the standards of care are being introduced.

Make a friend of your doctor. Try to save time by jotting down beforehand the questions you want to ask. If they are numerous, ask in advance for an extended consulting time. It may help to take a partner or friend along with you. Try to become a specialist in asthma by reading all you can (including the other chapters in this book!). If you have stress-related problems, or suffer from depression, make sure these are discussed.

If you cannot obtain all the answers you need, then you should ask for a referral to an asthma specialist at the local hospital. If you simply cannot get along with your G.P., you may change. Your chemist will give you the address of the local Family

* Dr Helman has listed the questions a patient *wants* to ask as: 'What has happened?', 'Why has it happened?', 'Why me?', 'Why now?', 'What will happen if nothing is done?', 'What should I do about it?'

Practitioner's Committee, who will supply a list of general practitioners, and may suggest someone with a special interest in asthma and hay fever.

The community nurses

All community nurses, in the U.K., have a vital role to play in helping patients and parents to manage their asthma successfully. *Health Visitors* take over from the midwife and have a special responsibility for children up to five years of age. They can help diagnose asthma in the first place and then monitor treatment. The role of the *School Nurse* has been examined in Chapter Nine.

District and *Practice Nurses* have the same responsibilities, except that the former work within a defined community and the latter only within a practice (which may cover many communities). They can receive special training at the Asthma Training Centre. When suitably trained, community nurses can run asthma clinics, either at community health centres or in general practice.

An individual nurse's role will depend on his or her experience. At the very least, it will extend to recording peak flow readings and teaching inhaler techniques. When suitably qualified, the nurse will in addition take a full history; suggest a treatment plan for consideration by the G.P.; teach self-management on a step-by-step system; set up regular reviews and give advice where needed.

The Asthma Training Centre

This was set up in February 1987 to provide special training in asthma for nurses of all kinds, but especially nurses working in general practice. Nurses spend the first six months studying a learning package at home, then spend two days at Stratford-upon-Avon to sit for a diploma and receive further instruction. As I can testify, having attended one of the earliest courses, the venue could not be more pleasant and Shakespeare's comments on life in general were an added evening bonus. The Training Centre can supply clinic record cards and a schools teaching pack, among other materials.

Other sources of information

The retail pharmacist

People who are worried about their medicines often fail to realize that their local dispensing chemist is not only well versed in the possible side-effects but also is very willing to explain what these are, as well as the purpose of the medicines and the correct way to take them. Medicines to relieve asthma and hay fever are among those most commonly prescribed, and the pharmacists can attend refresher courses on their use. If you ask them when you present your prescription they will add a note on the label as to function and purpose.

Pharmaceutical companies

All the leading suppliers of medicines used in asthma and hay fever have Medical Information Departments. These were set up to advise health professionals but are increasingly being used by patients who write or telephone asking about the treatments they have been prescribed. Telephone numbers are given under 'Useful Addresses' at the back of this book. If you live outside the United Kingdom, your retail pharmacist will advise the address of the local suppliers.

Regional Information Centres

These are being set up, under a Government initiative, by the fourteen Regional Health Authorities in the U.K. They not only provide answers to medical questions, often in the form of folders of information drawn from their extensive files, but will also deal with queries as to the local services that are provided. They can be reached by dialling (free) 0800 66 55 44 from anywhere in the U.K.; this number will be answered by the appropriate Regional Information Centre.

Self-help societies

These have been set up in many countries. Addresses are given in Chapter Seventeen.

The work of the National Asthma Campaign (U.K.)

A problem shared is generally reckoned to be a problem halved. The National Asthma Campaign currently has close to 200 branches, large and small, in the United Kingdom. It exists to help people with asthma and their carers to share their experiences and to learn from specialists. At the time of writing, annual membership costs £5. Half the members belong to branches.

The branches hold meetings which are open to the public and are addressed by doctors and other health workers. They distribute leaflets on many aspects of the illness, for example 'Take Control of Asthma' and 'Asthma in the Under-Fives'. *Asthma News* is published, in colour, four times a year and has a circulation of around 40,000 copies, bringing up-to-date information about treatments and current political issues concerning allergy. Video and audio tapes are also available, on loan. The Junior Asthma Club has its own newsletter.

Some branches organize Swim Groups, others provide dry-land exercises. Activity holidays are arranged for children with asthma, who gain thereby a great increase in self-confidence. The branches also raise money for research, in addition to central fund-raising, and currently the grants amount each year to just under £2 million. This supports research around the country, including two professorial chairs, each with teams of specialist scientists.

The National Asthma Campaign lobbies politicians, and was recently successful in making peak flow meters a prescribable item. There is an Education Committee which tackles such issues as asthma in schools, asthma in teenagers, and the development of self-management plans.

In October 1990 the **Asthma Helpline** was set up. By dialling 0345 010203 between 9 a.m. and 9 p.m. on a weekday, you can obtain – for the cost of a local call – advice from specially trained nurses on any problem connected with asthma or hay fever. In the first eighteen months, 10,500 calls were received, 9,000 about medicines and 5,500 to do with asthma in children. Any unusual questions are referred to the appropriate expert for comment, or are passed to a local branch of the Campaign if information about local medical services is needed.

In time of need

There are various ways in which people with chronic severe asthma, or those looking after them, may be able to alleviate real financial hardship caused by the illness. These are liable to change; 1988 Supplementary Benefit was replaced in the U.K. by Income Support. This eliminated some of the extra payments for which asthma sufferers might be eligible and for single payments substituted the Budget Fund which, for example, provides loans to enable people to buy equipment.

If you need information about any of the D.S.S. benefits, write to your local office. Local Authority social workers will be able to tell you what additional benefits can be provided from local government sources. The system as a whole will be explained by your Citizens' Advice Bureau. The broad categories of benefit currently are those set out on the following pages.

Asthma may disable for a time and then diminish; this presents a barrier to claiming some of the benefits, and persistence may be needed to obtain them. In the United Kingdom additional help may be obtained from the following:

Welfare Rights Officers at Town & County Halls

Community Health Councils (see local telephone directory)

Disabled Living Foundation, 380 Harrow Road, London W9 2HU (Tel. 071–289 6111)

Disability Alliance, Universal House, Wentworth Street, W1 7SA (Tel. 071–247 8776) publishes a comprehensive guide.

Action for Sick Children, Argyle House, 29 Euston Road, London NW1 2SI (Tel. 071–833 2041)

The Dept of Social Security's leaflet F 62 'Which Benefit?' is an essential guide. 'Sick or Disabled' is also helpful. There is a free telephone advice service: 0800 666 555 (also in Chinese -252 451; Punjabi -521 360; Urdu -289 188; Welsh -289 011). Charterline is a guide through the maze of services, for the cost of a local call on 0345 203040.

Benefit	Qualification	Leaflet number
Statutory Sick Pay	up to 28 weeks, paid by employer	NI 16
Invalidity benefit	pension after 28 weeks' sickness	NI 16A
Severe Disablement Allowance	for people of working age with 80% disablement	NI 252
Disability Living Allowance	help with getting around and personal care	
	under 65	DS 704
	over 65	DS 702
Invalid Care	for looking after invalids and not able to work	FB 31
Industrial Injuries	illness due to conditions at work	NI 6

Benefit	Qualification	Leaflet number
Disablement Benefit	which affect all the workers	
Disablement Benefit	for a prescribed industrial disease, such as occupational asthma	NI 257
Social Fund Benefit	a loan, repayable over 12 months, for equipment due to the illness	SFL 12 SB 16A
Income Support	when unemployed or sick	IS 20
Help with payment for medicines	an exemption certificate signed by doctor	P 11
	medical costs abroad	SA 29
	help with sight tests	GL AV
Pre-payment	prescription season ticket obtained from the Family Health Service Authority	FP 95
Local Authority		
Miscellaneous	Based on needs, not means. Varies from one local authority to another e.g. bus passes, telephones, adaptation to homes, nurseries, play groups.	
Housing Benefit	For people who need help with rent	RR 1
Council Tax	If on low income, or if house has been adapted for asthma, you may get a reduction	CTB 1

The orange-badge parking scheme

People with severe and persistent asthma find that mobility is greatly helped by the use of a car but in our crowded cities they may be concerned that they cannot park near the shops or services, or even close to their own home.

The Orange Badge Scheme, in the U.K., is designed to 'help people with severe mobility problems' by allowing them to park close to shops and public buildings, without being wheel-clamped unless causing an obstruction. The badge must be displayed with a parking disk showing the time of arrival. Holders can park without charge or time limit at parking meters and for up to three hours where yellow lines are in force. This does not apply to bus lanes. The national scheme does not apply to central London.

Badges are issued by the Social Services department of the local authority. To qualify there are various categories. As far as asthma is concerned, the relevant one is that you must have 'a permanent and substantial disability which causes inability to walk or very considerable difficulty in walking'.

Life insurance premiums

Some life policies include clauses that are restrictive to people with asthma, or load the premiums. You should admit to having asthma, since non-disclosure could be a ground for non-payment. However, there are insurance companies which take a modern view and do not load for people with asthma. It is a good idea to shop around.

PART FOUR

Complementary Medicine

CHAPTER FOURTEEN

Complementary Medicine

Changing attitudes to medicine

In Shakespeare's time, illnesses were treated by infusions made from plants as approved by custom or the herbals. Apothecaries existed in the towns; but they did not receive their charter until 1607, shortly before Shakespeare's death. In our own times, the apothecary's remedies are provided by a science-based industry which spends countless millions on research, while herbal remedies, another growing industry, are shunned by the orthodox doctors. We do, of course, take infusions of tea and coffee, but these were unknown to the Elizabethans.

It may at first seem that 'scientific' and 'local' medicine have grown far apart. Their differences can be over-emphasized, however. Many of the drugs used for treating asthma derive from plants used as remedies in ancient times. A few miles from where I live, the search continues. At the Brompton Hospital, a team has been investigating the leaves of the Gingka Biluba tree, used by the Chinese for thousands of years as a remedy for chest disorders.

Some would question whether the procedures of modern science are fundamentally different from those of 'primitive' medicine-men: both proceed by trial and error; both try in ingenious ways to render the toxic elements inactive while keeping their beneficial properties; both depend on the trust and faith of the recipients; both use esoteric language to describe the mysteries of their craft. There is, however, one big difference. Orthodox medicine draws its conclusions from very carefully controlled trials in which the active drug is tested against a placebo (a substance which is inert) not just on a handful of patients but on many. In contrast, the evidence in support of unorthodox medicine tends to take the form of anecdote, stories of individual cases which have not been studied in a strictly scientific way.

The advantage of using a 'double-blind' study, with half the patients on a dummy drug or 'placebo' (see page 84) and half on the active drug, is that in both cases the patient is equally susceptible to the power of suggestion. This can be very strong, especially where a bond has been established between the physician and the patient. In the double-blind trial, both patient and physician remain ignorant as to which is the dummy and which is the drug under trial.

Can 'alternative' medicine help people with asthma?

There are at least 130 alternative systems for treating our human ailments and many of these aim to treat respiratory illnesses. Few of the books which describe these remedies provide anything resembling proofs that they are effective. This is not surprising, since many of them were established long before modern science took over our civilization. They survived through the centuries because, for one reason or another, they made people feel better. It is only in the last year or so that a serious scientific study of these disciplines has been initiated, and the conclusions will not become known until the turn of the century. This is in contrast with the vast amount of evidence, from both clinical and laboratory studies, that orthodox treatments do work, especially where severe, life-threatening attacks are concerned. So until there is hard scientific evidence that alternative medicine can provide better results it should be used not as alternative but as **complementary** medicine. Seen in this light, alternative procedures often have the approval of conventional practitioners. It is, however, a good idea to consult your orthodox doctor as to the suitability of any system you may wish to try before you undertake a course of treatment.

A non-orthodox consultation may have its advantages. In *Living With Allergies*, Dr John McKenzie has written:

Alternative therapies are comforting, and a visit to a therapist is generally going to be a pleasant, soothing experience, which is rarely true of visits to hospitals or surgeries . . . The emphasis of many alternative therapies is to treat the whole patient on many levels simultaneously, with the final aim of reaching the point where the patient can maintain good health unaided.

Some complementary systems described

Acupuncture

This is a fully developed system of medicine, practised in China for over 3,000 years, which rests on a view of life which supposes that the whole universe is ruled by the interplay of 'Yin' and 'Yang'. These are opposing forces which have to be kept in balance when they operate within the body. If one organ is stimulated, then another will be sedated; and the balance will also be affected by universal forces such as the weather.

To a Western mind, this may at first sound strange and even absurd, until you recall that an illness such as asthma is swayed by shifts in the balance between the sympathetic and the parasympathetic autonomic nervous system; and any person with asthma will assent to the idea that the weather plays an important part in the ups and downs of the illness.

Western medicine does recognize that an organ which is diseased can produce pain at a distance and uses this to help diagnosis; but in Chinese medicine it provides a basis for treatment, which takes place at the surface. The Chinese believe that there is a kind of life force or 'Chi' which flows through channels, which they call 'meridians', beneath the skin. They think that the force can be redirected by stimulating acupuncture points, which lie along these pathways. In modern practice, the stimulation is carried out with long, thin, disposable, stainless-steel needles, a process which has been described as almost painless. The needles are inserted to a depth of between a fraction of an inch and two inches, and sometimes they are rotated between the thumb and forefinger.

These life-force channels have not been identified by Western medicine, but neurologists accept that acupuncture can sometimes produce prolonged relief from pain. One theory is that the pressure points can release the body's own pain-killing substances, the endorphins, which resemble morphine and heroin, and the body's own hormones. Another theory is that acupuncture blocks nervous impulses transmitted from the spinal cord. A third idea is that acupuncture makes use of the body's electrical fields, which can affect every human cell. That the fourteen channels or 'meridians' exist is not doubted by Chinese practitioners. It is possible for electricity to pass through a substance without changing it and to find its own pathway which does not depend on any that we can directly observe. The pathways have been explored by Chinese professors in various ways. One is by percussion, which generates waves that pass along the meridians; another is by electrical impedance, or resistance, at various points; a third is through radio-active tracers; a fourth, the measurement of local temperature. All these investigations point to the same pathways. This still does not explain 'how it works' – but then orthodox medicine does not understand how aspirin works!

This area of speculation is fascinating, but our immediate concern is whether acupuncture can help the asthmatic. To treat asthma the acupuncturist tries to control the 'Chi' through one or more of four meridians: the lung meridian, the bladder meridian, the heart meridian, the colon meridian; and the point of the ear can be used as well. An acute attack, mild or severe, would be treated, and swiftly relieved, by applying the needle to the 'Ding Chuan' point, just below the neck, and to other points which are referred to by a Chinese name or code (for example, 'Feishu' is Bl 13, or the thirteenth point along the bladder meridian). In China, relief from asthmatic spasm is seen as only a preliminary, and the aim is to control the asthma on a permanent basis without the need for any medicines. Any lesser state would be seen as 'crippling'. For establishing control on a longer term, that is, reducing inflammation and hyper-responsiveness, additional points would be used such as 'Lieque' (Lung 7). Hay fever and rhinitis can be eliminated, it is claimed, by adding two more points: 'Yintang' and 'Yingaxiang'. Not many controlled trials have been published. In a recent trial in India using forty-two patients, the best results were achieved with those asthmatics whose asthma was mainly allergic and of comparatively recent onset and where there was no dependence on steroids.

The sceptic may ask how the acupuncture points have been determined in relation to any particular illness. The acupuncturist will reply that they have been established by trial and error, and the evidence has been amassed by the Chinese universities, whose research teams can draw on the results of large numbers of treatments carried out each year, running into millions if all illnesses are considered.

One of the fascinating aspects of acupuncture is that diagnosis depends in part on the taking of pulses along the radial artery below the wrist, not just one pulse but as many as half a dozen where a really skilled Chinese practitioner is concerned. Blood travels along the artery in waves; by taking the pulse at, say, three points along its course, on the underside of the wrist, the character of the waves can be determined. If stronger at one of the three points than at another, the system is seen to be out of balance and will need correcting until the pulses are even. The pattern of these wave rhythms helps determine the diagnosis.

There are about 5,000 acupuncturists in Europe, but only a few hundred in the United Kingdom. The address of an Acupuncture Association which keeps a registry will be found under

'Useful Addresses', along with other addresses relating to complementary medicine. As far as asthma is concerned, the patient will attend every week until between five and ten treatments have been carried out. A return visit will be made if the symptoms reappear. Orthodox medicines can be taken, but the aim of treatment is to reduce dependency on them. Scientific proof that acupuncture can replace orthodox medicine is not available.

Clinical ecology

On the shelves of leading stationers and booksellers there are few paperbacks which provide an objective account of allergy but many which rest entirely on a subjective approach and which are plentifully supplied with *individual* case histories, designed to promote confidence in the method. Many are written by 'clinical ecologists', who claim that 'modern' foods are responsible for a wide range of complaints, ranging from swelling ankles and asthma to tinnitus and the consequences of vitamin deficiency.

No attempt is made to establish a link between a particular symptom and a particular food, or to use conventional challenge tests. Instead, unusual or bizarre procedures are employed, such as applied kinesiology, iridology, hair analysis, provocation-neutralization tests, Vega tests and electrokinesis. There is no scientific basis for any of these procedures.

Herbal medicine

Many preparations used in orthodox medicine to treat asthma were derived, ultimately, from plants. The difference between orthodox and herbal medicine is that in the orthodox kind the active ingredient has been identified and isolated; in herbal medicine, either the whole plant is used or a part in its entirety. In defence of this non-selective system it is argued that the plants often contain secondary substances which may make the effective ingredient either stronger or safer.

It is one of the principles of herbal remedies that if possible they should be based on local plants, preferably gathered at an appropriate time of day, because the chemicals in plants change from hour to hour. It follows that many herbalists grow the plants they need in their own gardens. As an example of this principle, there have been reports of asthma being dramatically improved when local unstrained honey has been swallowed, presumably because it has reduced sensitivity to some of the local pollens.

The aim in choosing a remedy is not, as in conventional medicine, to block any of the body's reactions but to treat the patient as a whole and to stimulate the body's own defences. In asthma, however, the treatments are usually anti-spasmodic and are used in conjunction with the orthodox bronchodilators, at least in the early stages. The doses are small – but not homeopathically small – and side-effects are rare. Of concern to orthodox doctors are those imported remedies which contain steroids in excessive amounts. The herbs used to treat asthma often have beautiful names, such as celandine, elder flower, fennel, hyssop and valerian.

One of the advantages of herbalism is that the practitioner does not simply prescribe a herbal remedy but takes a very detailed history, in the expectation that the underlying causes can be tackled at source. This history goes back to childhood, and great attention is paid to diet, lifestyle, exercise and breathing technique. As far as diet is concerned, the herbalists distinguish between what they see as acid-forming foods and acid-binding foods. The former include meat, cheese, cereals and nuts and are believed to increase the production of mucus in the airways. The acid-binding foods are thought to diminish mucus; they include fruits, root vegetables, milk, cane sugar, coconut and oysters. Since the turn of the present century, herbalists have advised people to keep separate those foods which need different digestive enzymes, and to take them at different times, broadly distinguishing between proteins (which, they say, leave acid residues) and cereals (which leave alkaline residues). The advice does not rest on any scientific basis and was challenged soon after it first appeared.

Homeopathy

This claims to be a complete system of medicine which rests on the principle that 'like can cure like': the idea that a substance which can produce certain symptoms in a healthy person at a large dose can, in a sick person, relieve those same symptoms when given in a tiny dose. This principle can be illustrated by an example. In the early nineteenth century, a certain Dr Hahnemann noticed that a large extract of Cinchona bark produced symptoms like those of malaria. This suggests that a dilute extract can stimulate the systems in the body which fight disease in much the same way that vaccines are used nowadays in immunization.

What seems to defy scientific logic is that the strength or 'potency' of a homeopathic remedy increases as the dilution increases. This dilution can consist of taking a tenth part of a solution of the substance in water or alcohol and by 'succussion' shaking it vigorously with ten parts of the diluent, and so on for as many as thirty dilutions. By the time the thirtieth succussion has been completed there may remain in the solution not a single molecule of the original substance. Homeopathic practitioners sometimes try to explain this in terms of modern physics, which tells us that it is energy and not mass which lies at the heart of matter and that it is possible for the energy of the diluent to be greatly increased by each successive dilution and for the water or alcohol molecules to be changed. This energy, it is suggested, can stimulate a response at the level of our body cells.

Of greater interest to asthma sufferers is the question, whether any of these remedies can relieve their symptoms. Like herbalists, the homeopathic doctors are interested in the possible triggers for asthma or hay fever; many are also qualified in orthodox medicine and prescribe conventional and homeopathic medicines at the same time. So it may be difficult to decide which of the three approaches contributes most to any improvement. The following case has been described: a girl of four had severe asthma which, over two years, did not respond to any of the inhalers. At the homeopathic clinic, skin tests showed a strong allergic reaction to house dust mite extract. The homeopathic doctor prescribed a homeopathically prepared solution of house dust and, at the same time, persuaded the mother to buy a solid foam mattress with a plastic cover and provide terylene pillows. Subsequently, after one dose of the homeopathic preparation, the symptoms of asthma disappeared and no more medicines of any kind were needed.

A third principle of homeopathy, which may puzzle anyone who believes (as I do) that asthma is not an illness of nervous origin, is that the choice of homeopathic remedy is determined not only by the illness but also by the type of personality or 'constitution' that is being treated. Rather in the same way that the ancient Greeks identified people as having 'humours' which made them phlegmatic, choleric, melancholic or sanguine in temperament, so the homeopathist decides whether the patient is independent or gregarious, tidy or untidy, anxious or confident; the type of asthma is also considered. Thus a patient who complains of night asthma and who has a restless and anxious spirit is treated with Arsenicum. Calmer patients with night asthma are more likely to respond to Ipecac. If the patient is sweet-tempered and affectionate and dislikes stuffy rooms, then Pulsatilla is tried. Ipacac is preferred if there is a copious production of phlegm, whereas if the asthma is dry or there is pronounced wheezing, then the therapist is likely to prescribe Spongia or Bryonia. If the asthma is easily provoked by emotion, especially anger, then Chamomilla is considered, and this is also used in children whose asthma makes them irritable.

This view – that asthma is linked to types of personality – is not generally shared by psychiatrists. The opposite view – that asthma may profoundly affect the personality – is easy to accept and this does perhaps support the notion that a study of the personality can throw some light on the severity of the illness.

Homeopathy is practised by some 300 medically trained doctors in the United Kingdom, who are also qualified in orthodox medicine and use both systems in conjunction. The homeopathic medicines are available under the National Health Service and there are six homeopathic hospitals within the service. The Faculty of Homeopathy is legally recognized; and both the present Queen and her father, George VI, have been patrons of the Royal London Homeopathic Hospital.

Treatment is given in the smallest doses that will bring relief. In an attack of asthma they will be given every 10 minutes, then every 15 minutes, with an increasing interval of time until a dose given once every 24 hours is reached. Constitutional remedies may need to be taken only as a single dose. Quite startling changes may be experienced, but these are not toxic effects and the medicines can be regarded as safe, cheap, easy to take, taste-free and capable of being stored for long periods. It is possible that the changes are due to the 'placebo effect'.

As with the other complementary medicines, an official Commission is investigating the claims of homeopathy and by 1999 will decide whether these remedies can continue to be prescribed on the National Health Service.

Hypnosis

The aim in hypnosis is to increase a patient's acceptance of the treatment proposed and to achieve a greater degree of relaxation before an attack. The patient can be persuaded, under hypnosis, that the autonomic system will function normally and not (as in asthma) swing too far towards the parasympathetic side of the autonomic pendulum. Hypnosis goes back to the Greeks and the Druids, but its fame in Europe dates from the 1760s when Franz Mesmer gave dramatic and sometimes hilarious demonstrations of his powers.

The way hypnotism works is as follows: the hypnotist persuades the subject to fix the eyes on an image such as a revolving wheel. The eye-muscles become fatigued and the eyes close. The therapist then talks in a slow, monotonous voice and suggests that the patient relax until a trance-like hypnotic state, somewhere between sleeping and waking, is achieved. Most people can be hypnotized and reach the stage of believing that what they are told will happen, provided that this is not at variance with their personal code of conduct.

Hypnosis will not relieve an attack already under way, but there have been cases in which it has helped asthmatics to achieve a state of calm relaxation when the wheezes first appear and so avoid a serious attack. Patients can be taught how to put themselves into a trance and practise 'auto-hypnosis' when they feel an attack coming on. Hypnosis can also help smokers to give up their habit. It is essential to use the services of a therapist who is also trained in orthodox medicine; a list of such practitioners can be obtained from the British Society of Medical and Dental Hypnosis (see 'Useful Addresses', page 287).

Manipulative therapies

Osteopaths remind us that, in the long history of evolution, Man has only recently walked on two feet with an upright posture. We put loads on the discs between our vertebrae which they were not originally designed to bear and, in our upright state, the organs hang down in an abnormal way. This can, under strain, set up stresses at the point where muscles attach to bones, and these can be painful if the affected area is close to a nerve. Osteopathy can free the tissue from strain and permit a better flow of blood not only to the nearby organs but also to more distant parts of the body.

This has some relevance to asthma, because the nerve supply to the lungs comes through the spinal cord and manipulation can remove abnormal strains that bear upon this nervous pathway.

The osteopaths also believe, as do physiotherapists, that people with asthma tend to breathe using the muscles of the chest rather than the diaphragm, and also to breathe through the mouth. This, as we have already seen, can contribute to the asthmatic response, and it can be corrected. Osteopaths are also concerned with the patient's environment and way of life as a contributing factor.

Chiropractors also pay great attention to the musculo-skeletal development and posture of the patient. After careful examination, backed by X-rays, the chiropractor will release joints between the vertebrae and the ribs to improve chest movement and stimulate the nerve supply to the muscles involved in breathing, including the diaphragm.

Qualified osteopaths and chiropractors, those who are registered by their national associations, have undergone a rigorous training covering the same pre-clinical sciences as orthodox doctors, but specializing in muscular and skeletal anatomy, in which their understanding is likely to be profound. It is still (in 1993) legal for anyone to set up, without training, as a manipulative therapist; only a registered practitioner should be consulted (see Useful Addresses, page 287).

Reflexology

This is a very old system, which in ancient China was used in conjunction with acupuncture. The principle is that, by deeply massaging certain parts of the body, beneficial effects are produced elsewhere. In the West, practitioners concentrate on the feet, not in the way chiropodists do, but because it is believed that very specific parts of the feet relate, in some mysterious way, to distant parts of the body, including the lungs. As the therapist gently strokes the surface, pain is felt in the 'sensitive area' and this, together with a crystalline feeling to the touch, shows where the deep massage should take place. Deep massage is carried out with the edge of the finger or thumb, in a circular motion. Orthodox medicine cannot detect any nervous pathways which might connect the feet with the internal organs in this very specific way, but the system can claim successes, including relief from asthma. The foot is very well represented in the brain and this may be a clue to the route by which the stimulus is transmitted. However, in the absence of controlled trials, a 'placebo effect' cannot be discounted.

Yoga

Yoga is now practised by many people in the West as a means of achieving both suppleness and relaxation and is a very old discipline, stretching back at least to 3000 B.C. Over the years many different forms have developed, often centred on a guru (one who dispels darkness). The aim has been to explore all the bodily functions and use correct breathing and posture to prevent or cure disease.

Each posture consists of a movement of the body, a mental state and a control of breathing. Breathing is especially important. Slow and controlled breathing, when it has been achieved, creates a state of calmness and is conducive to meditation. Highly disciplined teachers can reduce their breathing rate to two breaths a minute or raise it to sixty times that rate, at will.

Can yoga help people with asthma? A study has been reported in the *British Medical Journal* in which a sizeable number of asthmatics were treated with yoga in addition to conventional medicine. Compared with the controls (people who had only the medicines) the asthmatics had fewer symptoms and needed fewer drugs. The authors of this report looked for a reason and wondered whether yoga may have dampened the 'parasympathetic response', which causes a narrowing of the airways. What can be said with certainty is that yoga is the most profound way in which to learn relaxation.

Surprisingly, there is no register of qualified practitioners, but some local authorities include yoga classes in the programmes of their adult institutes.

Mind, body and spirit

Underlying much (but not all) alternative medicine is the notion that while orthodox doctors treat the body, and psychiatrists treat the mind, old-fashioned healing is also concerned with the soul or spirit. This supposes that soul or spirit exist apart from the body. However, I recall reading Gilbert Ryle's *The Concept of Mind*, when studying philosophy, and concluding that if you take away one, at the same time you remove the other! They are distinctions of language, not of substance.

PART FIVE

Appendices

CHAPTER FIFTEEN

The Questions People Ask – and Where in the Book to Find the Answers

Among the many questions people ask about asthma, there are some that crop up with great frequency. The cross-references following the questions are to the page numbers of this book where the answers will be found.

Symptoms and signs

'How do I know it is asthma and not bronchitis?' Pages 7, 177.

'Should I have a skin prick test?' Page 55.

'Is asthma a dangerous illness?' Page 10.

'When should I call the doctor?' Pages 136, 183.

Causes

'Are asthma and hay fever inherited?' Pages 37, 166.

'Are asthmatic people unduly nervous?' Page 242.

'Why is asthma often worse at night?' Page 76.

'Can colds cause symptoms of asthma?' Page 75.

'Are asthma and hay fever always due to allergy?' Pages 9, 221.

'Can changes in the weather affect asthma and hay fever?' Pages 65, 222.

'Is asthma affected by air pollution?' Page 68.

Precautions

'Should I give up smoking?' Pages 70, 170.

'Should I try to eliminate dust from the bedroom?' Page 44.

'Do we have to get rid of the pets?' Page 51.

'My son has asthma and he loves games; should I let him take part?' Page 190.
'If we move somewhere else, will the asthma improve?' Page 73.

Worries about medicines

'If they are taken day after day, will the effectiveness wear off?' Page 87.
'Can I become addicted to the medicines?' Page 83.
'Can I take too much relieving medicine?' Pages 87, 92.
'If I take more than one medicine, will this increase the side-effects?' Page 83.
'Do I have to go on taking the medicines even though I have no symptoms?' Page 100.
'If the attack gets worse, should I increase the dosage?' Pages 136, 154.
'How do I know whether my child is using the inhaler correctly?' Page 113.
'My neighbour's friend has been advised to use a nebulizer.
Should I have one too?' Page 122.

No one understands

'I am not sure my doctor understands my asthma. What should I do?' Pages 5, 246.
'The teachers at school will not let my child use his inhaler when needed. What should I do?' Pages 188, 190.

What about the future?

'Will my child grow out of asthma?' Page 169.
'Should I have another child?' Page 166.

CHAPTER SIXTEEN

A Manifesto for Patients with Asthma

In 1993, the National Asthma Campaign (UK) published a Manifesto to draw attention to the needs of people with asthma and to promote the best practices among health professionals, employers and all those who have an impact upon the lives of people with asthma. By permission of the Campaign, the manifesto is here reproduced in full, with supporting quotations.

Guiding Principles for Health Care

People with asthma have the right to expect the best possible care from experienced and committed professionals; care being developed as a partnership between patients and health professionals. Such care should be given according to nationally agreed guidelines. (as published in Thorax 1993:48 S1–S24).

The way in which acute asthma attacks are managed frequently differs from national guidelines. R. G. Neville *et al.*, *British Medical Journal* 1993; 308: pp. 559–62

Good Communication

People with asthma have the right to expect

o clear written and verbal advice about their asthma which

highlights the signs that their asthma is worsening and explains what they should do in that event
- ample opportunity to express their expectations of treatment, their fears about the condition and the medicines used to treat it
- to be made aware of sources of additional information and support such as the National Asthma Campaign

At the time of diagnosis only 7 per cent of patients are given 'plenty of information'; nearly two-thirds of patients want more. National Asthma Campaign/Mori Poll 1990

In partnership with their Doctor

People with asthma have the right to

- select the best inhaler device for them
- monitor their own condition using a peak flow meter
- control their asthma by following an agreed self-management plan

Two out of three patients do not use their inhalers properly. J.J. Kemp, *Asthma* (1990), p. 27. D. King, *British Journal of Clinical Practice* (1991), Vol. 45, p. 4.

From their general practice

People with asthma have the right to expect

- general practices to adopt agreed policies for the management of asthma which promote a uniform approach to asthma management
- specially trained professionals to review their asthma management once a year. In the case of care being shared between G.P. and Practice Nurse, the nurse should have had appropriate recognized training

In an emergency

People with asthma have the right to expect

- their calls for help to be treated as urgent by all health professionals, especially G.P.s, Practice Nurses and Receptionists
- a swift response by an ambulance which is staffed with trained paramedics, and equipped with oxygen and nebulizers
- on arrival in Accident & Emergency, to be given priority in the triage system (which gives priority to the most ill patients)
- a follow-up appointment in hospital, asthma clinic, or at their local practice
- prompt communication between Accident & Emergency Department and G.P. or Practice Nurse

At Hospital

People with asthma have the right to expect

- referral to a hospital specialist whenever necessary
- to be seen by, or admitted under the care of, a Consultant in Respiratory Medicine. In the case of children, they should be seen by a Consultant Paediatrician with expertise in asthma
- effective communication between hospital doctors and their G.P.

If admitted under a non-respiratory specialist, the person with asthma is less likely to receive steroid tablets, less likely to have their preventative treatment increased and as a result may be ten times more likely to be readmitted in the subsequent year than if their first admission was under a respiratory specialist. C. E. Bucknall *et al.*, *Lancet* (1988), vol. ii, pp. 748–50.

Research

People with asthma have the right to expect

- sufficient funds to be made available for research into the causes, prevention and treatment of asthma, and into finding a cure

The Environment

People with asthma have the right to

- breathe clean, smoke-free air at home, at college, at work, on public transport and in all public places
- smoke-free accommodation in universities, hostels or prisons
- daily information about air quality to be readily available at a local level

Passive smoking causes difficulty for 57 per cent of people with asthma. National Asthma Survey, 1991 (61,234 respondents)

There are only 9 stations in the UK which monitor all types of air pollution. Friends of the Earth

At school

Children with asthma have the right to expect

- easy access to their medication. Most children should be allowed to carry their own inhaler (with the possible exception of the very young)
- their school to have a policy on asthma and a member of staff who is responsible for that policy
- their school to be visited by a school nurse or health visitor who has received special training in asthma

93 per cent of school teachers do not feel that they know enough about asthma in children. Bevis and Taylor, *Archive for the Disabled Child* (1990), vol. 65, pp. 622–5.

At work

People with asthma have the right to expect

- equal employment opportunities, regardless of diagnosis, in any occupation commensurate with their abilities
- all employers to have a smoking policy which recognizes that passive smoking is a serious health hazard, and an established trigger for asthma

41 per cent of people with asthma are restricted in the work they do. Almost one in ten are forced to change their job because of asthma. National Asthma Campaign Poll, 1992

As a Consumer

People with asthma have the right to expect

- that insurance companies adopt an up-to-date approach to asthma and respect the benefits of long-term treatment
- legal protection against extravagant claims about clinically untested consumer products and scare-mongering advertising
- that governments should legislate against such medically misleading claims and call upon the Advertising Standards Authority to respond promptly to complaints about misleading advertisements. Such products should be submitted to the same form of evaluation as that required of medicines

CHAPTER SEVENTEEN

Useful Addresses

The following were checked in 1993, but may have changed since.

Self-help societies (U.K.)

National Asthma Campaign, Providence House, Providence Place, London N1 0NT (Tel. 071-226 2260) (see page 251)

Asthma Training Centre, Winton House, Church Street, Stratford-upon-Avon, Warwickshire, England, CV37 6HB (Tel. 0789 296974) (see page 249)

Action Asthma, P.O. Box 230, Bradford, West Yorkshire BD7 1BR
Educational material

British Lung Foundation, 8 Peterborough Mews, Parsons Green, London SW6 3BL (Tel. 071-371 7704)
This is concerned with research into all respiratory illnesses.

National Eczema Society, Tavistock House East, Tavistock Square, London WC1H 9SR (Tel. 071-388 4097)
Educational material

The Skin Treatment and Research Trust ('START'), Westminster Hospital, London SW1P 2AP (Tel. 071-828 7740)
Advice on skin contact allergy

Health Education Authority, Hamilton House, Mabledon Place, London WC1H 9TX (Tel. 071-387 9528)
Help for smokers wishing to give up

A.S.H., 109 Gloucester Place, London W1B 3PH (Tel. 071-935 3519)
15 branches in the U.K. providing help for smokers

Nutrition Advisory Service, Safeway Stores, 6 Millington Road, Hayes, UB3 4AY
Useful free booklets on additives

Carers' National Association, 20–25 Glasshouse Yard, London EC1A 4JS (Tel. 071-490 8818; Helpline: 071-490 8898)

Self-help elsewhere

Asthma Society of **Ireland**, 24 Anglesea Street, Dublin 2 (Tel. 001 716551)

Federal Council of Asthma Foundations Inc., **Australia**.
A.F. of Victoria: 101 Princess Street, Kew 3101 (Tel. 853 5666)
A.F. of Queensland: 51 Ballow Street, Fortitude Valley, Queensland 4006 (Tel. 252 7677)
A.F. of Tasmania: 82 Hampden Road, Battery Point, Hobart, Tasmania 7004 (Tel. 23-7725)
A.F. of N.S.W: 82–86 Pacific Highway, St Leonards, NSW 2065 (Tel. 906 3233)
A.F. of Western Australia: 61 Heytesbury Road, Subiaco, W. Aus. 6008 (Tel. 382 1666)
A.F. of South Australia: 341 Halifax Street, Adelaide, S. Aus. 5000 (Tel. 223 7235)
A.F. of Northern Territories: P.O. Box 40456, Casuarma, N.T. 0811 (Tel. 22-8817) and
Gregory Terrace, N.T. 0970 (Tel. 52-9219)

Asthma Society of **New Zealand** P.O. Box 1459, Wellington, New Zealand (Tel 499-4592).

The Wellington Asthma Society is at P.O. Box 11–159, Wellington (Tel. 384-4100)

In the **U.S.A.** the Asthma and Allergy Foundation can be

reached in Washington, D.C., on Tel. 202-466 7643; The American Lung Association, at 1740 Broadway, New York, on Tel. 212-315 8700; the Asthma Care Association of America in New York on Tel. 212-288 5416; the American Academy of Allergy and Immunology (611 East Wells Street, Milwaukee, Wisconsin) on Tel. 414-272 6071; the American Allergy Association is at Menlow Park, P.O. Box 7273, California 94026; Mothers of Asthmatics Inc. are at 3554 Chainbridge Road, Suite 200, Fairfax, Virginia 22030-2709.

In **Canada**, the Canadian Lung Association is at 75 Albert Street, # 908 Ottawa, Ontario (Tel. 613-237-1208). They have up-to-date addresses of provincial associations. At present these associations are: Alberta (Tel. 403-482-6527); British Columbia (Tel. 604-731-4961); Manitoba (Tel. 204-774-5501); New Brunswick (Tel. 506-458-2787); Newfoundland (Tel. 709-726-2550); Nova Scotia (Tel. 902-443-8141); Ontario (416-864-1112); Quebec (Tel. 514-596-0805); Saskatchewan (Tel. 306-343-9511); Yukon (Tel. 403-667-7462).

The Lung Association (national office), 1900 City Park Drive, Suite 508, Blair Business Park, Gloucester, Ontario, KLJ 1A3, is the secretariat of a network of asthma organizations. This includes those listed above, and the Asthma Society of Canada, 130 Bridgeland Avenue, Suite 425, Toronto, Ontario; also the Asthma Allergy Information Association, 65 Tromley Drive, Suite 10, Etobicoke, Ontario, M9B 5Y7.

Pharmaceutical Manufacturers (U.K.)

Allen & Hanburys Ltd, Stockley Park West, Uxbridge, Middlesex UB11 1BT (Tel. 081-990 9888)
Supplier of Ventolin, Becotide, Beconase, Flixotide, Flixonase

Astra Pharmaceuticals Ltd, Home Park Estate, Kings Langley, Herts WD4 8DH (Tel. 0923 266191)
Supplier of Bricanyl and Pulmicort

Boehringer Ingelheim Ltd, Ellesfield Ave, Bracknell, Berks RG12 8YS
Supplier of Atrovent, Duovent and Oxivent

Fisons plc, Pharmaceutical Division, 12 Derby Road, Loughborough, Leics LE11 0BB (Tel. 0509 611001)
Supplier of Aerocrom, Intal & Tilade

3M Health Care Ltd, 3M House, Morley St, Loughborough, Leics LE11 1EP (Tel. 0509 611611)
Supplier of Filair and Autohalers

Napp Laboratories Ltd, Cambridge Science Park, Milton Road, Cambridge CB4 4GW (Tel. 0223 424444)
Supplier of Phyllocontin & Uniphyllin

Medical Equipment Manufacturers (U. K.)

Advanced Technologists Ltd, Royd House, 224 Hale Road, Altrincham WA15 8EB (Tel. 061 903 9293)
'Alprotec' water-vapour-permeable covers for containing house dust mite allergen

Allerayde Ltd, Queens Head Court, 42 Kirk Gate, Newark, Notts NG24 1AB (Tel. 0636 613444)
Dust-control products, including water-vapour-permeable covers, and 'Allersearch' acaricide

Clement Clarke International Ltd, Airmed House, Edinburgh Way, Harlow, Essex CM20 2ED (Tel. 0279 414969)
Mini-Wright peak flow meters

Dunlopillo U.K., Pannal, Harrogate, North Yorks HG3 1JL
Latex foam mattresses

Ferraris Medical Ltd, 26 Lea Valley Trading Estate, Angel Road, Edmonton, London N18 3JD (Tel. 081-807 3636)
Peak flow meters

W. L. Gore & Associates (UK) Ltd, Churchgates, Church Street, West Woking, Surrey GU21 1PJ (Tel. 0483 756615)
'Intervent' water-vapour-permeable covers for containing house dust mite allergen

Lycam Ltd, Bieldside, Lucklaw Road, Balmullo, Fife KY16 0AY (Tel. 0334 870253)
Liquid nitrogen applicators for killing house dust mites in carpets and bedding; your hospital may assist

Medic-Aid Ltd, Hook Lane, Pagham, West Sussex PO21 3PP (Tel. 0243 267321)
Portable nebulizer, large-volume spacers and masks

Medic-Alert Foundation, 12 Bridge Wharf, 156 Caledonian Rd, London N1 9UU (Tel. 071-833 3034)
Steroid warning bracelets and necklaces

Medivac Healthcare Products Ltd, Bollin House, Riverside Works, Manchester Rd, Wilmslow, Cheshire SK9 1BE (Tel. 0625 539401)
Specialized vacuum cleaners

Medix Ltd, Medix House, Main Street, Catthorpe, Lutterworth, Leics LE17 6DB (Tel. 0788 860366)
Lightweight nebulizer

Slumberland plc, Salmonfields, Oldham OL2 6SB (Tel. 061-627 0133)
'Health Seal' beds to contain mite allergen

Vitalograph Ltd, Maids Moreton House, Buckingham MK18 1SW (Tel. 0280 822811)
Peak flow meters

Vorwerk (UK) Ltd, Unit A, Toutley Road, Wokingham, Berks RG11 1QN (Tel. 0734 794878)
Vacuum cleaners with zero escape of airborne house dust mite allergen

The Low Allergen House

This will be exhibited at the 'Future World Exhibition' in Milton Keynes, England, in June and July 1994.

Hosby Sales Ltd, Unit 24, The Nursery, High Street, Sutton Courtney, Near Abingdon, Oxon OX14 4UA
Supplier of Danish wood-framed houses which include tem-

perature and humidity control systems and air purification, and which can incorporate heat exchange units

Hosby can also suggest air exchange units to be fitted into existing houses and flats

Complementary medicine

Acupuncture Association and Register, 34 Alderney Street, London SWIV 4EU (Tel. 071-834 1012)

British Homeopathic Association, 27A Devonshire Street, London WIN IRJ (Tel. 071-935 2163)

They can supply a list of homeopathic doctors and many publications

National Institute of Medical Herbalists, 9 Palace Gate, Exeter, Devon EXI IJA (Tel. 0392 426022)

Osteopathic Medical Association, 22 Wimpole St, London WIM 7AD (Tel. 071-323 4810).

British Chiropractic Association, 29 Whitley Street, Reading, Berks RG2 OEG (Tel. 0734 257557)

The Association for Voice Movement Therapy, 7 Ballards Lane, London N3 IUX

CHAPTER EIGHTEEN

Further Reading and Special Acknowledgements

This book has been based mainly on talks given to three branches of the National Asthma Campaign, in West London, by scientists, consultants and practitioners who have made a special study of asthma and hay fever. These have included Professors Peter Barnes, Jonathan Brostoff, Tim Clark, Robert Davies, Charles Fletcher, Sean Hilton, Barry Kay, Tak Lee, Anthony Newman-Taylor, John Price, Neil Pride, Philip Snashall, John Warner and John Widdicombe, and Doctors Anne Cockcroft, Joe Collier, John Collins, Richard Fuller, Bill Frankland, Anthony Holden, Donald Lane, Bryan Lask, Michael Rudolf, Michael Silverman, Bonnie Sibbald, Jill Warner, Derek Williams and Nicola Wilson. The simplified approach to the cell biology has been based on talks by Professor Margaret Turner-Warwick.

One of the advantages of these talks has been the discussions, with patients and parents, which always followed them, revealing common concerns and queries.

Some of the paperbacks

The bookshops offer many titles which deal with allergy. Only a few are based on a scientific approach to the subject and many assume that diet is the only answer. However, there are some excellent paperbacks in the booksellers' lists, if not on all the shelves.

Asthma and Hay Fever (Dr Allan Knight, Dunitz, 1981) is a little out-of-date but he understands the family's concerns.

Asthma the Facts (Drs Storr and Lane, Oxford, 1987) is a goldmine of medical information, a classic of its kind, and one of the few books to tackle the emotional aspects. *Asthma at Your Fingertips* (Levy, Hilton & G. Barnes, Class Publishing, 1993) answers comprehensively all those questions which keep cropping up. *Conquering Asthma: an Illustrated Guide to Understanding and Self Care* (P. Barnes and Newhouse, Harcourt Brace, 1993) by two distinguished professors of medicine is much more concise than the title suggests, and is lavishly illustrated in colour.

Serious paperbacks on allergy include: *All about Asthma and Allergy* (Morrow Brown, Crowood, 1990); *Allergy the Facts* (Davies and Ollier, Oxford, 1989); *Living with Allergies* (McKenzie, Penguin, 1987). *Allergy? Think about Food* (Susan Lewis, Wisebuy, 1986) is a lay guide through the minefield of food triggers. A hardback which deals with 500 questions, *Allergies: Questions and Answers* (Rapp and Frankland, Heinemann, 1976), is out of print but may be in your library.

Books on complementary medicine do not devote much space to asthma or hay fever. A readable introduction to the subject as a whole is provided by A. Stanway, *Alternative Medicine*, Penguin, 1980).

Asthma News (The National Asthma Campaign) has been a source for many of the ideas I have incorporated. It can be obtained by becoming a Member (postal or branch) of the National Asthma Campaign, U.K.

CHAPTER ONE *Living with Asthma*

Page 12: Asthma in times past – I wish I had space to quote further from Dr Sakula's fascinating paper: 'A History of Asthma' (*Journal of the Royal College of Physicians of London*, Vol. 122, No.1, Jan. 1988).

CHAPTER TWO ***Why Some People Have Asthma***

Page 15: The quotation is from a slim but stimulating paperback, *Adult Asthma*, by Prof. Clark (Churchill Livingstone, 1984). In this chapter I have drawn on *A Practical Approach to Asthma* by Pawels and Snashall (CBA Services, 1986). Dr Geoffrey Laurent provided me with an insight into cells.

Page 26: pollen grains and mast cells. The diagram has been derived from *Food Allergy* (Edsall Publications).

CHAPTER THREE ***The Invisible Triggers***

Page 43: the Low Allergen Garden was created by garden designer Lucy Huntingdon, and botanists, gardeners and allergists contributed to the ideas.

Page 45: Dust that builds on dust. The diagram has been adapted from *Asthma in Childhood* by Professor Milner (Churchill Livingstone, 1984).

Page 46: War on the house dust mite. The practical measures are based on *The control of allergens of dust mites and domestic pets* by Coloff *et al.* (*Clinical & Experimental Allergy*, vol.22, Supplement 2, September 1992).

Page 65: Voice therapy deals with grunts and groans in a systematic way. It is explained by Paul Newham in *The Singing Cure* (Rider). See also page 287.

Page 67: Why thunderstorms cause asthma. Dr Jon Ayres' account of the Birmingham thunderstorm was reported in *Asthma News* (December 1987).

Page 68: Fog and filthy air. Friends of the Earth have been a useful source of information on pollutants.

Page 79: This table is based on a similar table in *Allergy*, a textbook published in 1993 by Gower Medical Publishing.

CHAPTER FOUR ***A Wide Choice of Medicines***

Most of the information in this chapter has been obtained from the pharmaceutical manufacturers.

Page 102: Sodium cromoglycate. A history of the discovery of

Intal has been written by Dr Suschitzy and published in *Chem. Britain*, vol. 21, 1985, p. 554.

Page 109: the Gallup survey was commissioned by Fisons.

CHAPTER FIVE *A Closer Look at the Inhalers*

I am indebted to the pharmaceutical companies for permission to reproduce or adapt drawings published by them. The drawings of a nebulizer on page 123 have been taken from a leaflet published in the past by the National Asthma Campaign.

CHAPTER SIX *Adjusting the Treatment*

Page 130: Four case histories. The case histories have been derived from a course for nurses run by the Asthma Training Centre at Stratford-on-Avon.

Page 136: What to do if things go wrong. This useful summary has been taken from a booklet by Dr Douglas Jenkinson, for use by his patients in a trial supported by Allen & Hanburys Ltd, with their permission.

Page 140: Posture during an attack. The illustrations are based on drawings in a leaflet devised by the physiotherapy department of the Royal Brompton Hospital, London.

CHAPTER SEVEN *The Patient Takes Control*

One of the first papers which showed that patients' perceptions of their asthma, based only on the symptoms, could be at variance with the actual state of their lungs, as revealed by measurement of expiratory peak flow, was written by two Australian doctors (Rubinfield and Pain) and published as 'Perceptions of Asthma' in the *Lancet*, 1976, pp. 822–4.

Page 143: The invaluable peak flow meter. The way in which peak flow readings can guide practitioners has been developed in *Asthma: the Management in General Practice* by Dr Ian Gregg (Update Publications, 1985). The charts used in this section have been taken from 'Peak Exploratory Flow Meter Measurement in the Management of Asthma', an excellent booklet devised for general practitioners in 1986 by Allen & Hanburys Ltd.

Page 154: Action plans: a guide to self-management. The plans, and the plastic cards, were developed by Professor Richard Beasley and colleagues in the Wellington Asthma Research Group, New Zealand, and were issued, in 1993, by the National Asthma Campaign (see Useful Addresses, above, and ask for booklet No. 7, 'Self-management and peak flow management').

Page 158: The measurement of success. This chart, and the commentary, have been adapted from a summary of a lecture by Dr Mark Levy which I wrote for *Asthma News* (February 1993).

CHAPTER EIGHT ***Living with an Asthmatic Child***

The best short introduction to this very important topic is *Childhood Asthma* by Professor Neill Buchanan, of Sydney University (U.K. publisher: Judy Piatkus, London, 1987). It includes, rare in medical literature, cartoons which are both humorous and sympathetic. I have drawn on a monograph for general practitioners ('Asthma in Childhood', by Dr Michael Silverman, Current Medical Literature Ltd, 1985).

Page 175: Avoiding the triggers. I am grateful to Dr David Hide of St Mary's Hospital, Newport, Isle of Wight, for providing an account of his trials

Pages 178–9: The Child's Asthma Card has been devised by the National Asthma Campaign, U.K.

CHAPTER TEN ***Living with Adult Asthma***

This has received less attention as a separate subject than childhood asthma. Professor Clark's useful book, *Adult Asthma*, has been cited above.

Page 198: How to recognize the degree of severity. This useful chart has been adapted from Professor Anne Woolcock's paper in the *European Journal of Respiratory Diseases* (vol. 69, 1986) and reproduced by permission of the publishers.

Page 200: the charts are from the Allen & Hanbury's booklet, cited above.

Page 202: Asthma in the 'Seventh Age'. The case histories have been taken from an article I wrote in *Asthma News*, August 1993. Shakespeare's famous account of the Seven Ages of Man was delivered by the melancholy Jacques, in *As You Like It*; 'Pipes and whistles in his sound' is a poetic description of asthma?

Page 205: The paint sprayer's tale was described by Dr Tony Pickering at the 1987 National Conference of the Asthma Society and reprinted in *Asthma News*.

CHAPTER ELEVEN *Living with Food Allergy*

My sources have included: 'Food Allergy' (Edsall Summary for Health Professionals No. 2, Edsall of London) and 'Food Intolerance and Food Aversion', a Joint Report of the Royal College of Physicians and the British Nutrition Foundation, *Journal of the R.C.P. of London* (April 1984). Introductions to the subject in paperback are listed on page 289.

CHAPTER TWELVE *Living with Hay Fever*

Books on asthma tend to pay little attention to hay fever, a notable exception being *Asthma and Hay Fever*, cited above, and the books which deal with allergies in a general way. I have drawn my material largely from excellent talks given to a West London branch of the National Asthma Campaign by Dr Bill Frankland, Professor Robert Davies and Dr Derek Williams. *Hay Fever: No Need to Suffer* by Johnson & Melville (Corgi Books) is good on ways of avoiding the triggers but is now out of date as regards medical treatment.

CHAPTER THIRTEEN *The Human Response*

Physicians concentrate on physical causes and on medical treatments, and asthma has not received much attention from psychiatrists. This means that one of the most distressing aspects of asthma and severe hay fever, the way they interfere with ordinary relationships, remains largely unexplored in print accessible to a lay reader.

In 1966 Dr Aaron Lask wrote, in *Asthma: Attitude and Milieu* (Tavistock), about psychological factors in asthma. In 1970, Drs Zealley, Aitken and Rosenthal published a paper in the *Proceedings of the Royal Society of Medicine* (vol. 64), in which they concluded a 'psychophysiological investigation' into patients with asthma and arrived at the view that we are no more and no less neurotic than the rest of the population! (I wonder if the same criteria should be applied to people who are ill as are applied to people who are well, since we live in a different sort of world.)

Action Asthma (see Useful Addresses) has published the results of a 'Young Asthmatics' survey 1993.

In 1983 Dr Aas reported to a symposium in Oslo the view of his Children's Asthma and Allergy Clinic that play, carefully adjusted, is essential for children with severe asthma, providing it calls for an imaginative insight into what is possible. Mrs Elizabeth Bell, who kindly helped with the sections on physiotherapy in the present book, would certainly agree.

In *Asthma News* (No. 14, 1987), the way asthma affects family relationships was explored by Dr Bryan Lask. Readers are recommended to turn to *Asthma the Facts* (cited above) for Dr Anthony Storr's introduction, 'Asthma as a Personal Experience'. This is a moving account, by a renowned psychiatrist, of his own reactions to his asthma.

I am indebted to three mothers of children with asthma for supplying written notes: Marguerite Griffiths, Beryl Schirn and Selina Thistleton-Smith. Judith Steward supplied the interviews on page 234. In *Help Me, Mummy, I Can't Breathe* (Souvenir Press, 1987) Susan Sutherland has written a dramatic account of the ups and downs of life with a severely asthmatic child in a foreign country. I have not read any fictional accounts of asthma, but hope to obtain *Of Love and Asthma* by Ferdinand Mount (Mandarin, 1991).

June Sykes kindly provided an up-date of the complex U.K. welfare provisions on pages 253–4.

CHAPTER FOURTEEN ***Complementary Medicine***

A good introduction to alternative medicine has been cited on page 289. Dr Stanway (*Alternative Medicine*) provides an extensive reading list. Penguin also published *Homeopathy for Everyone* and *Acupuncture and Chiropractic* in their Health series. The various societies whose addresses appear in Useful Addresses (Chapter Seventeen) will be able to suggest additional reading material.

In June, 1988, a famous article appeared in the prestigious journal *Nature*, in which a French team claimed to have demonstrated that a homeopathic solution could change other substances in contact with it. In the following month, a team investigating the methods used in the test threw doubt on their validity, but in an inconclusive manner!

I am indebted to Dr Anita Davies, Mr P. J. Cousins and Mr M. Hutchinson for descriptions of homeopathy, acupuncture and chiropractic respectively.

Index

Technical terms are defined as they appear